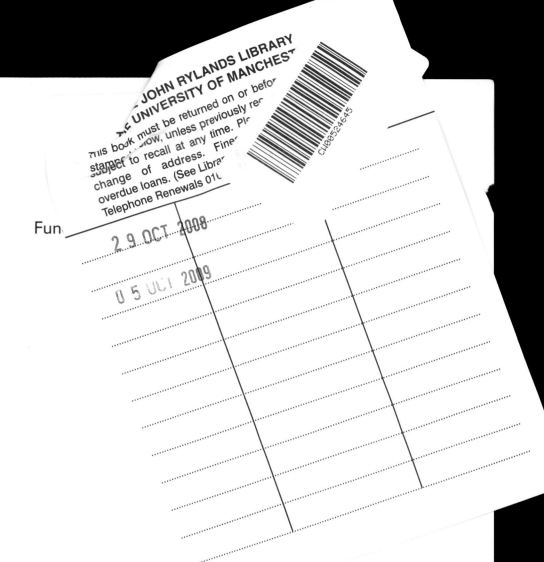

**Other titles in the Fundamental Aspects of Nursing series include**:
*Adult Nursing Procedures* edited by Penny Tremayne and Sam Parboteeah
*Caring for the Acutely Ill Adult* edited by Pauline Pratt
*Complementary Therapies for Health Care Professionals* by Nicky Genders
*Gynaecology Nursing* by Sandra Johnson
*Legal, Ethical and Professional Issues in Nursing* by Maggie Reeves and Jacquie
    Orford
*Men's Health* by Morag Gray
*Tissue Viability Nursing* by Cheryl Dunford and Bridgit Günnewicht
*Palliative Care Nursing* by Robert Becker and Richard Gamlin
*Women's Heath* by Morag Gray

Series Editor: John Fowler

**Other titles of interest**:
*New Ways of Working in Mental Health* edited by James Dooher
*Forensic Mental Health Nursing: Interventions with people with 'personality disorder'*
    edited by the National Forensic Nurses' Research and Development Group
*Palliative Care in Severe Dementia* edited by Julian Hughes
*Legal Aspects of Consent* by Bridgit Dimond
*Legal Aspects of Patient Confidentiality* by Bridgit Dimond
*Legal Aspects of Medicines* by Bridgit Dimond

**Other books edited by John Fowler**
*The Handbook of Clinical Supervision – Your Questions Answered*
*The Handbook of Practice Development*
*Case Studies on Practice Development*
*Staff Nurse Survival Guide*

**Note**

Health care practice and knowledge are constantly changing and developing as new research and treatments, changes in procedures, drugs and equipment become available.

The author and publishers have, as far as is possible, taken care to confirm that the information complies with the latest standards of practice and legislation.

# Fundamental Aspects of Community Nursing

*The experience of community nursing*

*Edited by*

## John Fowler

PhD MA BA DipN Cert Ed RGN RMN RCNT RNT

*School of Nursing and Midwifery,
De Montfort University, Leicester*

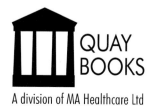

QUAY
BOOKS

A division of MA Healthcare Ltd

Quay Books Division, MA Healthcare Ltd, St Jude's Church, Dulwich Road, London SE24 0PB

British Library Cataloguing-in-Publication Data
A catalogue record is available for this book

© MA Healthcare Limited 2006

ISBN-13: 987 1 85642 302 1
ISBN-10: 1 85642 302 6

Printed by Gutenberg Press Ltd, Gudja Road, Tarxien, Malta

# Contents

# Preface

There is no theory–practice gap within the content of this book, as it is written by real people living and working in the real world. It is a book about experiences of what it is like to work as a community nurse, of being a student on a community placement and (most important of all) what it is like to be a patient in the community. Each chapter captures the experience of community nursing, and I am indebted to all the contributors who took time out of their busy lives to write an account of their experiences. When writing a nursing textbook it is quite easy to describe assessment procedures, theorise about interdisciplinary working and describe communication systems, but it is not so easy to portray the realities of assessment or working with other professions or the practicalities of planning care. The contributors of this book have really captured the realities not only of working in the community, but of being a student on placement. Central to all is the first chapter, by Nancy Telford, which gives you an insight into the realities of a being patient who lives day after day with a devastating illness.

Many books on community nursing will be structured on such themes as assessment in the community, managing care and multidisciplinary working; these topics are to be valued and as a student they will help you examine some of the core issues relating to community nursing. However, for me nursing is about the experience of caring, and this book captures how different nurses put that ideal into practice. Most of us learn from our experiences far more than we do from listening to a lecture. During your training it is unlikely that you will be able to spend time working with all of the different types of nurse that work in the community and hence gain that experience. However, this book allows you to enter into the vicarious experience of a number of specialist nurses. Helen McVeigh and Ruth Rojhan are both District Nurses, but each with distinct differences within their role. Ann Clements is an experienced health care assistant and gives you a wonderful insight into her role and perceptions of others. Zoë Wilkes and Helen Rhodes are both consultant nurses and function in very unique and different ways; as you read their accounts both of them will make you feel, 'I would really like to do that job'. The work of the Health Visitor is well portrayed by Karen Ford, who gives you a sample of how health education and health care practice can be incorporated into practice. Tony Scarborough's account of working as a therapist in mental health within GP surgeries is a fascinating description of how ordinary people's lives are often traumatised by relationship problems and of the way in which a mental health worker can intervene before the person's health becomes more seriously affected. The development of the role of the practice nurse has increased over recent years and Lindsey Wilkins' account gives you a flavour of the variety of interesting work that they undertake.

Much of the future development of health care will take place in the community. Health centres are increasing in size and in the variety of services that they offer to patients, often in a far more accessible format than attendance at large hospitals. There are considerable differences in running a 'one-person GP practice' to running one that has eight or more GPs, four or more practice nurses and a host of other facilities. This needs management and organisation, and Pat Brookhouse's account of being a practice manager gives an excellent account of the importance of having dedicated people managing practices.

Finally, there are the accounts of Stuart Ward and Sarah Hudson, who at the time of writing were third year students who had recently undertaken their community experience. Whilst the memories were still fresh in their mind they wrote their accounts of that experience. These are excellent accounts and capture the experience of being in the community and the sorts of nursing skills and knowledge they learned. They also give you their tips on how to make the most of the experience and also how to survive.

Finally, I have provided introductions and comments for each chapter. Originally I intended to write only a few sentences to set each chapter into context, but the lecturer within me took over and I found myself drawing out issues and hopefully challenging the way you think about and perceive community nursing. As you read all of these accounts you can process the information on at least two levels. Firstly, there is the appreciation of what each person is saying and the development of quite a broad understanding of different people's roles and abilities; this is very useful and will help you appreciate the wide role and responsibilities of community nurses. But there is a second level that requires deeper reflection and an unpacking of your previous views, perceptions and understanding about not only community nursing, but also the wider body of nursing and how you as an individual function.

What you are reading about in this book are accounts of what people do, what they believe in, and to some extent why they are doing it. This is a great privilege, because people are letting you not only into their working role but also into their beliefs aspirations, and implicitly into the way they think. If you can reflect on these accounts and on your own nursing practice in ways that really make you explore and challenge your beliefs and understanding, not only about community nursing but also about how you function as an individual, then you will learn some very powerful lessons.

John Fowler
*Principal Lecturer – Nursing, De Montfort University, Leicester*
*Education Consultant – Nursing, Leicester City West Primary Care Trust*

# Contributors

**Pat Brookhouse**
*Practice Manager; Postgraduate Certificate and Diploma in Health Services Management; Postgraduate Certificate in Medical Education*
Pat started her career as an invoice clerk in the pharmacy department of a large hospital. She continued her administrative career in the hospital, taking on greater responsibility and larger budgets as she progressed through the managerial ranks of the health service. She then moved into the community as a practice manager of a developing GP practice and has been an integral part of that team for a number of years.

**Ann Clements**
*Community Health Care Assistant*
Ann is an experienced health care assistant working in a community nursing team in Leicester. She commenced her work as a health care assistant working night shifts in a hospital setting. She soon realised that she liked the caring aspect of this work, and when her children were old enough to allow her a little more working freedom she applied for a job in the community, where she has worked for a number of years.

**Karen Ford**
*Health Visitor; RGN, BSc (Hons) Health Science; RHV Specialist Practitioner; BSc (Hons) Community Nursing; Extended & Supplementary Nurse Prescriber; Certificate in Intensive Care Nursing*
Karen worked for 20 years in secondary care, including being a sister in an intensive care unit, before becoming a health visitor. Following her training as a health visitor she worked in an inner city area and then in two different county areas. She was recently appointed Senior Lecturer at De Montfort University.

**John Fowler**
*Principal Lecturer – Nursing, De Montfort University, Leicester; Education Consultant – Nursing, Leicester City West Primary Care Trust*
John qualified as a general and mental health nurse in Portsmouth in the 1970s. He worked as a community psychiatric nurse before taking up a post as mental health nurse tutor. He then moved to Leicester as a general nurse tutor and has

continued to work there in a number of educational posts. He has published widely on a number of nursing subjects, and his PhD thesis was on experiential learning in nurse education. He currently has a dual post as principal lecturer at De Montfort University and education nursing consultant to Leicester City West PCT.

### Sarah Hudson
*Third year student nurse*
Sarah commenced her working life as a dental nurse and then moved into the national blood service as a venepuncturist and latterly as a team leader in that service. She then decided to become a nurse and commenced training at De Montfort University. At the time of writing she was in her third year of training and had just completed her community experience.

### Helen McVeigh
*RGN; BSc (Hons) Community Health Nursing; Nurse Prescriber*
Helen has spent 17 years working in the community. Her earliest experience of community nursing was as a student nurse knocking on the doors of her patients wearing her leather motorbike jacket! At the time of writing she was working as a district nursing sister in the busy inner city of Leicester. She has recently taken up a post of Senior Lecturer at De Montfort University.

### Helen Rhodes
*Consultant Nurse for Assist Service (a nurse-led primary care facility for asylum seekers); BSc (Hons) Primary Care Nursing; Practice Nurse Pathway; RN; RSCN*
Helen is one of those people who are always looking for new and challenging roles. She had a varied nursing career in the UK and then worked with the Aboriginal population in Australia. On returning to the UK she worked as a practice nurse. In 2000 she was appointed as a clinical nurse specialist with special responsibility for the new population of asylum seekers. This role developed, and Helen became the country's first consultant nurse for asylum seekers and has developed a service that is a model for other PCT and health care providers.

### Ruth Rojhan
*District Nurse & Practice Educator; RGN; DN; Cert. CPT; PG Dip (Ed); MA (L&T); RNT*
Ruth's first experience of community nursing was as a child during her school holidays, when she would sit in the car while her District Nurse mother did her nursing rounds. Following nurse training and varied clinical experience she started work as a community nurse and eventually became a district nursing sister and a practice educator, passing on her skills not only to student nurses,

but also to student District Nurses. Ruth is currently a Senior Lecturer at De Montfort University.

## Tony Scarborough
*Senior Practice Therapist; BSc; DPSN; RMN; ENB A12; ENB 603*

Tony qualified as a mental health nurse and worked in a number of in-patient settings. He then moved into the post of charge nurse for the community child and adolescent services where he worked for a number of years. He has undertaken a number of post-registration courses and now specialises in what are often called the 'talking' therapies. He was appointed Senior Therapist in the new primary care mental health service that aims to offer short-term therapeutic approaches based in GP clinics.

## Nancy Telford
*Person with Parkinson's (PwP)*

Nancy worked as a librarian in a busy sixth form college until the effects of Parkinson's disease forced her to retire. She is actively involved in supporting other people with Parkinson's disease and frequently advises her local Primary Care Trust on patient issues.

## Stuart Ward
*BA (Hons); MSSCh; MBChA; Third year student studying for a DipHE in nursing at De Montfort University, Leicester*

Following a degree in drama Stuart worked as a health care assistant while he was 'resting'! He then trained as a chiropodist, but missed the nursing approach that he had experienced as a HCA and decided to train as a nurse. At the time of writing he was a third year student, having just completed his community placement.

## Zoë Wilkes
*Nurse Consultant – Children's Palliative Care; Dip HE in Nursing – Child Branch; BSc (Hons) Specialist Practice Nursing (Child in Pain); MSc Allied Health Sciences*

Zoë trained as a children's nurse and worked in a children's ITU in London, gradually developing a 'vocation' for palliative care. She then worked in a children's hospice in Kent before moving to 'Rainbows', the Children's hospice in Leicestershire. She was then appointed consultant nurse for children's palliative care.

## Lindsey Wilkins
*Practice Nurse; RGN; RM; BA(Hons) Health Studies Specialist Practitioner (General Practice Nursing); Postgraduate Diploma Applied Health Studies*

Lindsey qualified as a general nurse and then as a midwife. She worked as a midwife for a number of years and then moved into the role of a practice nurse in 1989. During her experience as a practice nurse she has worked in a number of practices and seen many NHS initiatives that have impacted on primary care. She currently has a dual appointment in which she works as a practice nurse in a GP practice for part of the week and as a practice nurse adviser for Leicester City West PCT.

# CHAPTER I

# A plaint about Parkinson's disease

*Nancy Telford*

## Editor's introduction

In this chapter Nancy Telford tells her story of life with Parkinson's disease, which she has had for the last seven years. Nancy use to work as a librarian in a busy sixth form college, but due to her Parkinson's disease had to give up work four years after she was diagnosed. Nancy had a very full life as librarian, wife, mother, social activist, musician, part-time youth worker, holiday-maker, gardener and many other household and family roles, like those we all have. Now, as Parkinson's disease robs her of her physical expertise, she still maintains a very full life, but it is one that she battles with every day, often fighting the same battle but with different people.

When you or I speak, people listen and understand what we are saying, usually with no look of suspicion or hesitation. But when Nancy speaks the words can be a little slurred. This is the battle of communication – of not having to apologise for speaking in a slightly slurred way, of convincing people that although your speech may be a little slurred what you are saying is not only quite intelligent, but because of the effort it takes you to express your self, it is probably more thoughtful and 'intelligent' than the words of others who say the first thing that comes into their head. When you, as a professional nurse, meet Nancy it will only take you about 30 seconds to come to this conclusion, but for those 30 seconds Nancy has to fight that battle. Every time she meets someone new, be it a health professional, supermarket assistant, or a stranger in the street, Nancy will have to fight it again.

What about the battle of 'non-verbal' communication? One of the cruel effects of Parkinson's disease is the way it robs the person of the smile, the look of surprise, the frown – in fact, nearly all the subtleties that our facial expressions give us. So when Nancy is in a group or talking to her friends or children, they will not see the facial expressions that normally accompany our verbal communication and give it that quality of warmth and humour. Often what attracts us to another person is not so much what they say but how they say it, and it is these expressions that speak a language of their own. So Nancy has the battle of conveying warmth, humour and commitment to the people she is with, otherwise they will read her as uninterested, bored or simply not listening. This is a battle that is extremely hard to win day after day.

There are many other battles that Nancy fights each day. The battle of getting up when every muscle in your body just does not want to move, and when it does it is like moving a heavy weight. The battle of dressing, washing, going to the loo (at the appropriate time!). And that's before you get down stairs and start to think of breakfast.

As you read through Nancy's powerful account of her experiences and involvement with the health services, try to think what you can learn from her experiences. If you were to visit Nancy in the community you would knock on the door of her house, and she would then let you into her house but her home. Her home is full of her life. The photos, pictures, books, furniture – these will all be part of the life that this person is letting you into. So always remember how privileged you are to be allowed inside, not only this person's house, but her home and her life.

In her story Nancy uses the analogy of Parkinson's disease as a mugger, one that has attacker her and robbed her of precious parts of her life. However, this mugger is quite subtle. He does not take everything at once. When he first mugs her he does not take that much, but he keeps coming back. Nancy calls in the police to try to prevent the mugger doing more harm, but sadly the police are either too busy or just don't seem to be able to prevent him from coming back.

# A plaint about Parkinson's disease and the parlous state of the Health Service

Think of your health as wealth, health as money. Think of Parkinson's disease as a balaclava-ed mugger, sneaking up on you and your money. Parkinson's disease is a subtle mugger. It first steals minor capabilities like good handwriting or being able to hold a cup without shaking, or it turns the habitual expression of good will on your face into an unsmiling mask. Never mind – you still have £5 to see you through to the end of the week: your determination, your other compensatory skills which have your friends saying admiringly, 'You really can't see any bruises of where you have been mugged...'. This is termed the 'honeymoon period' of the disease, when I was able to work four more years after diagnosis.

Then the mugger begins to steal more valuable things, like your sense of balance and your free movement through space. Now you can't jive, pirouette, pivot, or play octaves in quick succession on the piano. Your confidence begins to shrink, ever so slightly, so you make ever more compensations to make sure you are still you. You join something and take excessive responsibility for doing something you really believe in (because who knows how much time you have left?), or you bury your head in levodopa until its power is stolen by the mugger. Either way, you've managed to lose even more of your wealth of health, until the mugger finally wins and you break a hip or catch pneumonia or your mind goes the way your mobility has.

This deprivation of yourself by Parkinson's disease can be devastating, but your impulse is (and it must be kept to fiercely): *not to let the mugger win*. Ways of outwitting it are many and various, but they need to be coordinated to achieve the end of a sane mind in a moving body, which dies of something else!

Now it is *possible* to be poor without feeling deprived (look at most of the Third World), but I *feel* deprived as well as poor with Parkinson's disease, because during the mugging of the last seven years, the 'police' (in this metaphor, the health professionals) have not got together and examined all the evidence and mostly seem not to be available to help me in my quest of living to outwit the mugger.

This is an account of my experience as remembered, so it's possibly not entirely accurate. It is an accurate record of how I feel, and even if the facts may have been a little different the result is the same. This is my perception of the illness, the effect that it has had on me.

# My diagnosis

This occurred very much at a GP level. My own GP was fortunately an excellent diagnostician. Although he had never seen much Parkinson's disease before, he said my description of my early symptoms was excellent and said it described in an almost textbook way the symptoms of Parkinson's. Following those initial early consultations he came around to our home after the diagnosis was confirmed and sat with my husband and me answering our endless questions as much as he could. My experience of receiving this initial diagnosis although a devastating blow, was delivered with humanity and expertise by a caring doctor. Sadly, however, this has not been the experience that a number of other people with Parkinson's have had.

Some people received their diagnosis in hospital, and were told, quite literally, 'You have Parkinson's disease', and given little or no information or support and then had to go home alone on the bus.

Someone else was told, 'You have Parkinson's disease. Retire and buy your own business since you are young'.

Another person, 'You have Parkinson's disease. There is little can be done – you'll just have to get on with it!'.

## Other people's experience of being diagnosed with Parkinson's disease

It's bad enough being mugged, but to see the 'police' almost as accomplices, is like being mugged by the people you go to for help. There is a right way to do it: the GP should refer a person with Parkinson's disease to a neurologist, preferably with a specialist interest in Parkinson's disease, and/or find the Parkinson's disease nurse specialist in the area. If at all possible they should be sent home to or with someone who cares! Tell them that *'There is much that can be done and that you will be pretty normal in the short to mid term'*. This little sentence would constitute about 100% improvement on what happens to many people. If they have younger children, tell them *not* to share medical dictionaries or Internet addresses with each other or with you, because they give the worst possible scenarios with graphic pictures. There is a time and place for this sort of information, but certainly for me it was not at this stage. I wanted to make as much of this strange honeymoon as possible.

## My early stages

This section centres on what I know and understand and what I need versus what a health professional knows and understands. I have read and now know a lot about Parkinson's. Sadly, I now know all about its probable causes, the avenues of research toward a cure, the way the brain is affected and the symptoms. I probably know more than most health care professionals, both from a theoretical perspective and certainly from an experiential one. However, what I often lose sight of is how to control the beast, so I need inventive, constant, monitored help in being consistent. Why has no one considered taking a baseline of daily activity to see when and how I improve or get worse? I need someone to follow up other methods of approaching the problem. I need for my notes not to be lost – three times in hospital, twice in appointments. I need to have regular physiotherapy, which is not available, to keep from developing attenuated muscles, or at least supervised exercise sessions to keep me strong against the mugger. As this is not available, I have had to start private physiotherapy sessions.

## My place, my care, your hospital

I would like the professionals in the health service to see me as a contributor to my own care. I need people in the health service to know how much I hate hospitals (as most of us do), because we see them as institutions that will take away all our individuality. It is almost as though they are trying to control us; it is like being in prison. To you they are your workplace and where you want to be; however, we regard them and you as scary, because you can reduce us just to ill people without status, instead of the efficient managers or housekeepers or lawyers that we are in real life. This is not a deliberate action on your part; it is the result of your knowledge and the necessary routines of hospitals, but most of all it is the result of our vulnerability. Read Erving Goffman's (1961) book on asylums to find out more about institutions. When I go into hospital I need to be left with my own drugs (or my carer needs to keep them) because they need to be taken according to symptoms, not according to drug routines on the ward. If I don't take them at the right time, I can become frozen and unmoving and unmoveable. If the doctor in charge doesn't understand the drug regime and writes down the wrong dose, I can start hallucinating like a friend did, trying to save his wife from the doctors, whom he saw as evil knights!

## My place, my care, my home

As for care in the community, I give a hollow laugh. Is this unfair? Not from my perspective. I've seen three different occupational therapists in three different uniforms, and they all said the same thing (although they were helpful concerning equipment). I've seen physiotherapists twice in my house, twice in hospital and four times privately. Do I need tell you who sorted out my foot pain in 2002 and then my leg pain in 2005?

I've have a wonderful speech therapist who was and is really helpful, and I've seen her about six times over the past seven years. Every six months I see the neurologist and he is primarily interested in how drugs are treating me, but he does not seem to have the time for, or interest in, how my life is. He listens patiently while my husband and I tell him about new drugs I can't have because the authority can't afford to buy them, and pooh-poohs most of the theories that we advance, sometimes in desperation, about what could make a difference. I do not feel able to talk to him in between appointments, but why am I complaining?

My condition has a nurse specialist: formerly Maddie and now, after no one was in post for a year, Jean. Maddie and Jean are both, in different ways, wonderful. They really listen, they really care. The trouble is, they have 3000 patients with Parkinson's disease on their caseload, so they can't monitor you or see you that often, and they have 25 telephone messages on their answerphones each day and why should I add to that pile? (Can you guess what happened to Maddie?) The new framework for people with long-term conditions says we get a holistic case management approach soon. I believe they think it's going to happen, but I don't think in fact it will. There isn't enough to go around – enough of anything – but mainly what are lacking are coordinated care at home, support for exercise and physical activity and monitoring of drugs. And the worst thing: now I'm an 'expert patient', the health service is making me look after my own condition. I've been well and truly mugged!

## Editor's comments

How did you feel reading Nancy's story? What can you learn from her experience? There is a theme of continuity of care: so many professionals all going in and asking the same questions, so many people with only a surface understanding of her disease and the implications that it has for her life. The experts, be they the consultant or the specialist nurse, seem to have so many other people to look after. Nancy, like many other people with long-term conditions, very quickly became the expert on her own condition. It is up to the professionals to use that knowledge, to build upon it if appropriate, at times to correct it if it is misinformed, but at all times to value it and the person who is at the centre of the problem. When you visit people like Nancy in the community, you see them on their terms. When they visit the professionals in hospitals, the positions are often reversed. The person feels disempowered, as Nancy expressed in her views of hospitals. Community care meets the person on home ground. It is important that we don't take that away from them by the use of language or the way we view or treat them. Nancy, like many people, is an expert patient, and we must treat her as such.

# Reference

Goffman, E. (1961) *Asylums: Essays on the Social Situation of Mental Patients and Other Inmates*. Anchor Books, New York.

# CHAPTER 2

# A student nurse's community experience

*Stuart Ward*

## Editor's introduction

If you are a student nurse reading this book prior to your community placement, try to collect your thoughts about what your expectations are. Now reflect upon how those views were developed and who influenced their development. Are they positive expectations, negative or a mixture of both? It is very important to realise how influential such expectations can be upon our attitudes and behaviour prior to our gaining our own experience of the situation. If you enter any new placement or new experience with negative expectations, then it will probably become a self-fulfilling prophecy that they are met. Likewise, if you enter any new placement or life experience with positive expectations, then you will probably achieve a positive experience. 'Believe in your self and believe in others' is a good attitude of mind to take you forward positively. This is one of the points that comes across strongly as you read Stuart's account of his community placement as a student nurse. There are a collection of other useful and interesting facts, not to mention the survival tips, but the strong undercurrent is this sense of being a positive learner.

# A student nurse's experience of community nursing

## My background

On completion of my school education in Louth, Lincolnshire, I studied for an actor–musicianship degree at The Rose Bruford College of Speech and Drama (Manchester University accredited). Following graduation, dwindling finances and numerous failed attempts at auditions prompted me to change my vocational direction. I gained employment as a care assistant at a private nursing home in Louth, where I worked full-time for four years, and enjoyed this experience immensely. Improved finances encouraged me to move on to develop my educational prospects. I discovered an interest in foot biomechanics, and so studied for a diploma in Chiropody at The Open College of Chiropody and Podiatry, Maidenhead, Berkshire. Upon qualification, I split my work as an independent domiciliary practitioner between Sheffield and Louth. Three years later, I had 'itchy feet' to get back to the nursing profession and broaden my skills. I was accepted at De Montfort University, where I am currently in my final year, preparing for life as a qualified nurse.

## My expectations of community nursing

'Community nursing: nothing but old people and leg ulcers – isn't it?' This was not an uncommon impression of what fellow students, non-related health professionals and (dare I say) some qualified nurses gave when I informed them of my forthcoming practice placement in the community. The last 18 months have taught me to be open-minded prior to commencing each placement, promoting a neutral and non-judgmental focus for which I incorporate enthusiasm and professionalism. I was not going to treat this placement any differently from my previous ones.

I was looking forward to community work because it would make a refreshing change from the hospital environment and I would not be expected to work long days or night shifts. On my first day, as I approached my placement medical centre, memories of those days when I worked as a domiciliary chiropodist flooded back and how I loved the inter-professional relationship between patient and practitioner. Conversation was not merely informal pleasantries, but often personal and sincere. I was, after all, entering someone else's private domain

– their space, their world, their history and on occasions their inner deep secrets. I was not just a chiropodist, but a spiritual listener, psychologist, trustee and friend. I would welcome these feelings of expressionism again in community nursing.

## My apprehensions and experience

Of course, I had some pre-placement apprehensions. For instance would I achieve a successful workable relationship with my allocated mentor? Would I settle into my working area? Would my car be safe? Would patients like me and trust me enough for me to implement therapy on them? Time would tell. In a hospital setting the student nurse is likely to spend ten weeks on either a medical, surgical or critical care ward. Three weeks into placement you gain a good understanding of how the ward is managed and adopt a routine of working that suits you. You witness patients coming and going and familiarise yourself with the drugs most commonly prescribed. You spend a day or so working with selected members of the multidisciplinary team and your nursing skills are continually repeated to demonstrate your capability to think and work safely in practice. After seven weeks, however, you are ready for a change of scene. In contrast, my ten-week placement on community passed so quickly, with each day differing from the next. The community nurse comes across as a universal practitioner who accommodates the services of both children and adults, providing therapy to medical, surgical, palliative and rehabilitation patients.

## My typical day

A day with my mentor commences around 8:30 a.m. The first two hours of the morning are likely to focus on patients with neurological deficits like multiple sclerosis, cerebral vascular accidents or acquired neurological trauma who need nursing intervention for their personal hygiene management and eliminatory habits. There are visits to insulin-dependent diabetics who are inefficient in managing their diabetes independently, who therefore require community nurses to draw up the prescribed units of insulin, monitor their blood glucose accordingly and ensure that they maintain compliance with their regimen.

From 11:00 a.m. to 12:00 a.m. the community nurse will run a clinic back at the medical centre, in which 12 or more patients will pass through the doors to have their ears syringed, sutures removed, staples extracted, or a wound cleansed for an infected ingrowing toe-nail or septic navel piercing, in addition to the administration of numerous vaccinations, from influenza to vitamin B12.

Between 12:00 a.m. and 1.00 p.m. the nurse is back on the road again, going to clients who require complex wound cleansing and dressing technique, usually as a result of post-surgical complications. Alternatively, this part of the morning may be set aside for patients requiring a continence assessment, or a urinal catheter maintenance review.

An hour's lunch break precedes our return to work at 2.00 p.m. The nurse starts the afternoon by visiting or re-visiting patients who need nursing intervention to assist their personal hygiene and bowel management. Time in the afternoon may be devoted to caring for individuals requiring palliative intervention or continuation of care, which could include the reassessment and implementation of care needs to accommodate the individual's present condition.

The community nurse will run a leg ulcer clinic two to three times a week which incorporates aseptic wound cleansing and wound dressing therapy. Ultrasonic Doppler assessments are frequently implemented to investigate vascular patency, followed by either intense compression bandaging, or referring patients to the hospital's vascular studies department for advanced investigation. Providing the paperwork is completed and filed, the day's work is accomplished by 5.00 p.m.

## Other opportunities

Whilst on community, there were many opportunities to partake in pre-organised activities, from bandaging and dressing techniques to continence, tissue viability, diabetic and palliative care workshops. I also visited a funeral parlour where the emphasis was on what support services were available to grieving relatives. During a visit to the British Red Cross, I was confronted by a warehouse full of provisions that could accommodate any individual, whatever their disability and whatever their need, from walk-in baths to a completely re-designed kitchen aimed towards maintaining a person's independence and quality of life.

As with any placement experience, the more you put into it the more you get out of it. If there was one particular learning experience I will take away from community, it is the value of careful preparation in referring hospital patients to community nurses. Whilst the community nurses are on their rounds, referrals are directly made via answerphone. During my ten weeks I experienced a relatively large number of messages that were extremely amateurish in content. Below is an example of some of the types of call received:

Err... hi, just letting you know that Mr Smith who lives at [address] will be discharged today. He... err... requires a wound check... err... following a recent hip operation. Could you... err... visit him between 9:30 and 10:30 this Thursday as he needs to be at the luncheon club for 12:00, many thanks.

This is by no means an over-exaggeration. I also dislike talking to an answering machine. I become vulnerable, insecure, forget what I want to say or how to say it, and all because there is no one on the other end of the line with whom I can engage in conversation. As a final year student working my last few months on a hospital ward, I am expected to effectively organise safe patient discharge. In order not to give the same amateurish impression, I have constructed a plan to assist me in making appropriate phone messaging referrals to District Nurses – see the box.

## My reflections on the community experience

I cannot recall any unhappy or discouraging moments. If anything, my time on community was a success. The staff were extremely supportive towards my learning development, whilst patients and their relatives made me feel very welcome with endless cups of tea and biscuits. Undoubtedly, my favourite period was being given the opportunity to go out and about independently on delegated care with a selective caseload, providing therapy to patients with whom I had built up a healthy rapport over several weeks. Though I was initially nervous, there was a determination inside me to do well, partly for my mentor, who had faith in me, and partly for the Primary Care Trust I was working for. Just as importantly, however, I wanted to prove to myself that I had the confidence and the initiative to make it as a professional nurse.

Before commencing therapy on a patient, I would take time to carefully read the client's nursing documentation. Reading the comments made by the nurse from the previous visit was important to identify whether therapy had changed, ceased to exist, or remained indifferent. On a couple of occasions that I recall, nursing implementation had altered with regard to wound cleansing procedures, and on a separate occasion a doctor had prescribed a topical medication to replace an existing one. Reading the nursing notes is like reading a recipe: providing you follow the instructions to the letter, you will provide safe practice. If in doubt, contact your mentor.

Being out in the wide world on your own, making important decisions for yourself, looking out for the welfare of your patient and taking their trust in your hands can be somewhat daunting. At the same time your nursing knowl-

# Making referrals to the community team

- Firstly, ensure that the patient's medical and nursing notes are with you prior to making the phone call.
- Ask colleagues not to interrupt your call.
- Ensure that your surrounding area is relatively quiet in addition to speaking clearly and slowly, as information can be easily misinterpreted if you are within a busy environment and speak with a soft, quick or abrupt voice.
- Introduce yourself as the nurse instigating the discharge, giving your full name and title.
- Name the hospital and ward from which the patient is to be discharged.
- Identify the ward's telephone number (including area code).
- Provide information with regard to:
  - Full name of patient, date of birth and sex.
  - Patient's full postal address and home/mobile phone numbers.
  - Patient's hospital number.
  - Patient's registered General Practitioner.
  - The date of planned discharge.
  - The date for when community nurses are required to make their first visit.
  - Patient's communicatory abilities and independent/non-independent factors.
  - Brief reference to patient's medical history.
- Explain:
  - Patient's presenting complaint.
  - What therapy the patient is presently receiving and with what tools.
  - Why the patient needs community intervention.
- Finally, ensure the patient is discharged with at least two visits' worth of therapy intervention, where applicable. For example, staple extraction: normal saline, dressing packs, gauze, staple extractors and Mepore dressings.

edge comes to the forefront of your mind. You realise that there is no room for error and that short-cuts are not an option; instead, a professional approach is adopted subconsciously.

# Making the most of the community experience

Below are some helpful points that successfully guided me through my delegated care:

- Talk to the patient. The student nurse has an opportunity, unlike in certain hospital settings, to communicate effectively with their patient. Ask them how they are; think holistically. If the patient wants to talk, encourage the discussion – you may after all be the only person they see until the next planned visit. This is a good opportunity for the student to develop skills related to confidence in conversation, engaging in eye contact and the ability to hold a conversation.
- If a patient appears unwell, or should she identify abnormal signs and symptoms to you, write it down in the patient's notes and report your findings to the named nurse (or your mentor) as soon as possible.
- Are there enough resources for the nurse to carry out practical procedures on the next visit, including dressings, aprons, gloves, dressing packs, steripods, cleansing-wipes, ointments, creams, paperwork? It can be time-consuming and frustrating and appear unprofessional when you do not have the appropriate provisions available.
- Following therapy, ensure that your written notes are dated and timed accordingly and what you are documenting is specific and to the point in relation to the procedure(s) performed. Write preferably in black ink, adopting legible handwriting. Sign and print your name clearly, so that it can be recognised by others.
- Show willingness and enthusiasm. Patients rely on you to motivate and improve their quality of life and well-being. They appreciate what you do for them, so be proud and enjoy your independence.

# Final thoughts

I would strongly consider applying for a job as a community staff nurse on completion of my diploma. I would want to apply for a position that provided a good preceptorship package, as I would need to build up the skills and knowledge required to work in a relatively independent way.

Once I returned to the wards following my community placement and declared an interest in this area, I was confronted by the myth that suggests that nurses become de-skilled when they venture out into the community. Personally, I disagree. I visualise nursing in the community as one large hospital that spreads itself over several miles. On a hospital ward I would be responsible for the care of at least ten patients on a bay, each with similar ailments according to the specialised area. On community I will be expected to be responsible for the same number of people, if not more, during each working day, the majority of which are likely to require different nursing interventions from each other. The type of nursing care delivered by community nurses is quite vast and may not reflect the experience of qualified nurses who had their student nurse experience many years ago.

I have not witnessed any evidence of the community nurse becoming de-skilled whilst out in practice. On the contrary, they perform the same jobs as would be expected on a hospital ward, such as holistic nursing assessments; cannula insertion; blood extraction; baseline observations; referrals to specialist teams; intravenous therapy; case conference participation; and care of a patient with a tracheotomy, stoma or naso-gastric tube; in addition to skills relevant to compression bandaging; palliative intervention; patient-centred approach to care with major carer/family involvement; and a good knowledge base with regard to computer literacy. These days, of course, there are numerous academic degrees out there to broaden the community/District Nurse's continual professional development.

Primary Care Trusts will soon be expected to offer people a host of services to their community, providing the investment is there to support them. The Government's introduction of the National Service Frameworks has been set out to reduce hospital re-admissions through health promotion and re-educational strategies, whilst holistic care will be provided to patients within their own home environment instead of a hospital. It could be argued that the role of the community nurse has never been more in demand.

## My survival tips

I have put together a list of pointers that helped me to progress successfully through my community experience:

- Carry a mobile phone (ensure you charge it up the night before) and insert the numbers of the nursing staff who are in the team for that day.
- Write down the telephone numbers of the patients you are going to visit just in case you get lost or stuck in traffic. Ensure that staff members have your number too.
- Give the staff a list of your patients, preferably in visiting order, and estimate a return time to base.
- Ensure that you write down the full name of the patient and correct house address prior to visiting. If patients have key-fobs, write down the number.

- Ensure that your student identification is on your person, particularly when visiting vulnerable patients and patients for the first time.
- Take time to familiarise yourself with the Department of Health's National Service Frameworks and the NHS Plan (Department of Health, 2000) in addition to digesting information relevant to your area's demographic and epidemiology background.
- On your travels take a pocket nursing dictionary and a *British National Formulary* in order to familiarise yourself with the numerous terminology and medications.
- Become confident in manual blood pressure technique prior to commencing your community placement. As part of a patient's assessment process or review, you will be expected to take manual blood pressures efficiently. Additionally, a fob-watch for pulse and respiratory monitoring is recommended.
- A small pad on which to scribble notes – very useful.
- A surplus supply of black and red pens.
- Quality dressing scissors are essential, especially when assisting to remove four-layer bandaging.
- A street map of your designated area.
- Make sure you keep your petrol (or local transport) receipts, and record your daily mileage. You may be entitled to make a claim for travelling expenses. And finally, good luck!

## Editor's comments

Stuart has given an excellent overview of his experience as a student nurse in the community. It is interesting to note that the 'message' that he received from a number of areas, prior to his placement, was that his community experience would be slow and a de-skilling experience. Stuart's experience was quite the opposite: it was a full and busy experience with considerable focus on actual nursing practice, with the development of a large number of essential nursing practices. Stuart demonstrated a mature approach to his learning. He was enthusiastic to learn and entered the area with a non-biased objective viewpoint. This paid tremendous benefits to his enjoyment of the learning experience; as he says, 'you get out of a placement what you put in'. Of all the useful information and tips that Stuart has included in his account, this must be the most important lesson for all students for all placements, and also for all qualified staff in all areas of work: the more you put in the more you will get out. Enthusiasm, commitment and genuine respect for your colleagues are wonderful qualities that, once developed, will help you to become a superb nurse.

# Reference

Department of Health (2000) *The NHS Plan: a Plan for Investment, A Plan for Reform*. Department of Health, London.

# CHAPTER 3

# A District Nurse's experience

*Helen McVeigh*

## Editor's introduction

Much of community nursing is carried out by District Nurses, but what exactly is it that District Nurses do? If you have already had a clinical placement in the community then you will almost certainly have spent time with a District Nurse and have gained a good understanding of their role. If your previous understanding of District Nurses came from television programmes, particularly those set in the past, you will probably have been quite surprised at a number of aspects of their work. The somewhat idealistic view of a homely lady riding a bike or driving a classic Morris Minor carrying a small bulging leather bag and discussing a particularly difficult patient with a somewhat patronising overweight GP is indeed a picture of the past. The modern District Nurse is part of a busy team, responsible for a large number of patients, many of whom have acute high-dependency needs. District nursing is a team approach led by a senior nurse in charge of the team who will have gained a post-registration qualification in community nursing at either first degree or masters level. This is the district nursing sister/charge nurse. Within that team there will usually be a number of registered nurses, usually between two and four. In addition, there are a number of health care assistants, usually between four and six.

Job satisfaction in the community is usually very high; this seems to be due to the independence, flexibility and personal contact with patients and their homes and families. It is often work that allows nurses to work around their own family commitments. The district nursing sister is normally full time, but it would not be uncommon for at least half of her team to work part time. Whilst this creates a few problems when people are off duty, there is not the same problem of maintaining patient continuity as with part-time staff who work in hospital wards. A nurse who works two days a week or four mornings a week can quite easily visit the same patients each week, and this tends to give part-time staff greater job satisfaction than they might get in a hospital setting.

Most nurses that work in the district nursing team are usually quite experienced, and a number have worked in their current role for a number of years. If you are a student nurse on placement with the district nursing team your first impression may well be of a group of somewhat 'mature' staff, particularly if you are only 20 years old! But do not be put off by this impression – some of the most dynamic, motivated and innovative staff I have ever met were in the district nursing team. So don't be off put if the coffee room conversation seems to focus on their children, gardening and the bargain buys at ASDA! These nurses and the patients that you will be meeting will help you learn very important aspects of nursing that you cannot gain from hospital wards.

To gain the maximum benefit from working in the district nursing team you will need to become an active learner. By this I mean that you will need to look at what people are doing, observe how they interact with their patients and their relatives and reflect on what is happening. Make sure you take every opportunity to discuss your observations with the staff you are working with, and ask them questions about how they deal with unusual situations. This is quite different from your ward placements. On a busy ward there is always something you can go and see. If one patient is sleeping you can go and watch or be part of a sterile dressing or medication round. But this is a more passive kind of learning: you just position yourself where the action is and it sinks in. In the community there is less 'action' happening around you; hence you have to seek out yourself what you can learn. So it is the ideal place to develop your relationship skills with patients, relatives and staff. Observe the different ways in which staff assess and consult with patients, the way they give reassurance, and the way they show empathy and care for their patients. Watch the experts, ask them questions.

District nursing sisters/charge nurses are team leaders. They are leaders, managers, clinical specialists, teachers, mentors, trouble shooters and policy writers, and in their spare time they make the coffee and do the filling. The following account is written by Helen, an experienced and dynamic sister who works in a busy inner city area. As you read through Helen's account, try to think how you would prioritise the various roles that she has. How would you lead a team, inspire them and support them when you only see them for an hour a day? The district nursing sister is one of the most rewarding roles in nursing; it combines expert clinical practice and leadership of a team, but it is also one of the most demanding roles. Is Helen's role one that you would aspire to?

# The District Nurse experience

The overall aim of a District Nurse's post is the management of the district nursing team and a community client caseload. The principal elements of the role are to plan, implement and evaluate high-quality research-based community health care practice to effectively meet the continually changing and evolving health needs of individuals, groups and communities. This requires effective coordination and liaison across the whole of the multidisciplinary team to provide high-quality effective holistic care to patients within the community.

The key responsibilities of the District Nurse's role are:

- **Managerial and professional practice**
  - Management of the nursing team
  - To utilise appropriate management skills and both provide and encourage leadership within the team
  - To utilise and contribute to health promotion strategies which promote health and prevent ill health
  - To liaise effectively across the multidisciplinary team
  - To effectively manage and utilise appropriate resources
  - Teaching and education of students and team members
- **Clinical and professional practice**
  - Management of client caseload
  - Plan, implement and evaluate evidence-based practice to meet needs of community/individual patients
  - Effective assessment of need
  - Effective utilisation of reflective practice

## My background

I have been a community practitioner for 17 years, a period spanning more than half of my nursing career. As a newly qualified staff nurse my aspirations were hospital-based and I did not envisage that a subsequent career pathway would lead to the community. My first experience of community nursing was a 12 week placement as a student nurse in inner city Birmingham, an enjoyable experience from which I remember the positive feelings of accomplishment that the responsibility of being entrusted with a small caseload of delegated patients to visit at the end of the placement conferred. However, at that time, as an impoverished student I drove a motorbike, and cannot imagine how many of these patients felt when answering the door expecting to find the student nurse and being greeted by an individual resplendent in protective clothing and full-face helmet on their doorstep.

The choice of working again in a community environment, once qualified, was taken primarily as a necessity as it afforded me the opportunity to work regular hours, which at the time fitted with family and home life. Embarking on a career as a community nurse, I initially worked on twilight and half-night shifts in the inner city. This had its own significant challenges, not least of which were developing a feline aptitude for nocturnal vision in map reading, and locating house numbers and doorbells in the dark. Although I had made the decision to work in the community largely to meet personal needs, I quickly discovered that working as a community staff nurse re-awakened those positive feelings from my days as a student, and realised that I enjoyed immensely this branch of nursing. Subsequent career development included working as a part-time community staff nurse in an inner city practice managing the treatment room and leg ulcer clinic. It was here that I developed a special interest in leg ulcer management and tissue viability, an element of practice fundamental to community nursing that I remain passionate about.

## How to qualify as a district nursing sister/charge nurse

In order to develop and progress as a community practitioner I chose to undertake further training to qualify as a District Nurse. Prior to 1996, District Nurse training had been at diploma level; however, proposals set out by the UKCC (1994) suggested that education in preparation for specialist practitioner should be at degree level. As a result I completed the newly implemented BSc (Hons) Community Health Nursing course – a 45-week full-time programme, 50% practice-based and 50% theoretical, a structure which supports recommendations that all specialised practice courses should have an equal division of theory and practice (Canham, 2002). The entry requirements for this programme require evidence of education to at least Diploma of Higher Education level and a minimum of two years' post-registration experience, and although not essential, community experience is beneficial. Although I enjoyed the challenge, the course was very intensive and my family was glad when I successfully completed and qualified as a District Nurse, partly because I reverted to sanity, but mostly because the dining room table reappeared from under a mountain of books and paper.

# The skills of a District Nurse

I believe proficiency as a community practitioner requires certain qualities and attributes, and the effective District Nurse needs to develop and utilise certain skills. Of primary importance are skills in communication – an ability to communicate effectively is fundamental to nursing practice and holistic health care delivery (Barr, 2001). Effective communication skills are required on many levels: on a one-to-one basis with clients, with team members, with members of the multidisciplinary team and across different agencies. Moreover, this may be via many different media: direct verbal contact, written notes and reports, telephone and email. The link for each piece of the jigsaw that ensures a community nursing team works well together is fundamentally efficient communication. District nursing also requires exceptional coordination and organisation skills and a good memory. My caseload may have in excess of 200 active clients at any one time, requiring coordination and planning of visits, a myriad of referrals and liaison with various primary care team members and other agencies. The uniqueness of the community environment for each practice area and each individual patient means that a District Nurse's ability to assess, interpret, evaluate and implement effective health care interventions cannot be underestimated.

# The responsibilities of a District Nurse

Each District Nurse is responsible for a team of community nurses and a caseload of patients. Typically a caseload comprises individuals requiring health-related interventions or support, either linked to specific general practitioners' (GP) practices or allocated geographically. My caseload is linked to four different GP practices in four separate surgeries, and consequently good communication and effective time management are essential. Although the community nursing service provides a 24-hour service, my hours of work are essentially Monday to Friday between 8:00 a.m. and 5:00 p.m., with weekends and Bank Holidays worked on a rotational basis. Due to the unique nature of community nursing the content of each day is almost always varied and different; however, the structure of each day usually follows a similar pattern.

Our district nursing team meets to coordinate the workload at the beginning and middle of each day. My first priority in the morning is to sort and filter the messages. Patients requiring visits are identified, contacted and prioritised according to need and the subsequent visits are delegated to staff members as appropriate. Referrals to the district nursing service come from a variety of sources (GPs, hospitals, residential homes, other agencies, carers, relatives or patients themselves) and are largely via brief telephone or fax messages. Consequently it is essential to clarify and confirm details. Time is a valuable resource, and I have on many occasions been greeted by bewildered individuals when attempting to locate patients from wrongly given addresses. One member of my team who was newly appointed only began to question the validity of the address she had been given when her mileage to one visit approached that of her normal total for the day! Early morning is when, as a team, we discuss issues relating to the workload for the day, and it allows team members to feed back on the patients on their caseload. Time for liaison is important – as the District Nurse I may not see members of the team until the next day, and although some of the team may meet after lunch to coordinate afternoon visits, a significant proportion of time is spent working alone, with communication limited to brief mobile phone messages.

Following the early morning caseload review, my day consists of a variety of tasks: visits to patients, meetings, report writing, case conferences and liaison with other professionals, agencies and members of the multidisciplinary team. Although I communicate with GPs through inclusion in regular (usually monthly) practice meetings, discussion of individual patients is often opportunistic and I will frequently seize the chance to pop into the consulting room between patients during surgery time. Like most District Nurses I have a good rapport with the GPs in my practice. The District Nurse may often have extensive knowledge about the chronically ill and/or housebound patients registered at the practice, and therefore the relationship between nurse and GP can be mutually supportive; effective exchange of information can enable a better quality of care for these patients.

A significant proportion of most days will be spent on holistic assessment of patients new to the caseload or on evaluation and review of existing patients. The District Nurse's expertise is in holistic assessment. To be effective, assessment should be founded on sound evidence-based practice. I would visit most new referrals often with students or less experienced staff, although some referrals would be delegated to experienced community staff nurses.

## Assessment in the community

The length of time taken to complete a holistic assessment can vary considerably, from 45 minutes to in excess of two hours, depending on its complexity. Assessment is a phased process:

■ **Preparation**: checking the referral, liaison with referee and arranging time of visit.

- **The visit**: assessment of the patient and identification of nursing needs, completion of patient-held notes
- **Implementation**: care plans and delegation of care, nurse prescribing, liaison with other agencies
- **Evaluation**: review of existing care and amendment

Typically I would use a nursing model as a framework to support the assessment process. It is important to use extensive communication skills throughout, allowing patients to express their needs in their own words and identify their own priorities, whilst skilfully guiding them into providing the information that will enable me to effectively plan care and identify actual and potential capabilities, and at the same time also including relevant health education and information. I will often find myself engaged in a discussion on anything from the latest soap opera news to the best recipe for chicken tikka, information which enables me to pick out relevant values and lifestyle and cultural influences. My interviewing skills are backed up by observational skills, interpretation of non-verbal clues and skills in identifying and interpreting risk. Moreover, I have to incorporate an understanding of elements such as family dynamics, psychological influences and patients' response to ill health. Often multiple health needs and problems are identified, and this entails establishing priorities and utilising other professionals and agencies where necessary. Although I endeavour to gain as much information as possible on the first visit, it is a cumulative process, with the team contributing as care is implemented.

## My typical caseload

The potential range of visits and identified care on my caseload will always be quite varied, which presents a significant challenge as a community practitioner to ensure that I have up-to-date evidence-based knowledge and awareness of a variety of illnesses, treatments and disease processes. Clearly this embodies the notion of lifelong learning and its relevance to nursing practice. I frequently liaise with other specialist practitioners (e.g. Macmillan, tissue viability, infection control, respiratory and hospital outreach nurses) to ensure that the care delivered is of high quality and to enable the team to meet the varied needs of clients whilst also ensuring they maintain safe and competent practice within current standards.

The range of patients on the caseload would typically include:

- people requiring post-operative wound care
- people with chronic wounds, such as leg ulcers and pressure areas

- people requiring simple procedures (e.g. administration of injections, eye drops or enemas)
- diabetic clients requiring administration of insulin or support in self-management
- people requiring management of chronic diseases (e.g. multiple sclerosis, renal failure, Parkinson's disease)
- people requiring management of malignancy/terminal care (palliative care and support and bereavement)
- people requiring assessment and management of continence problems

A significant proportion of cases will involve wound management and tissue viability issues, although these may also be part of a package of care implemented to meet multiple needs, particularly with older clients and those with long-term illnesses. Health promotion and health education are elements fundamental to any care package. Enabling patients to manage their own health can prevent subsequent ill health – for example, most diabetics on a caseload are encouraged in self-care and self-monitoring, with support, education and promotion of patient understanding as the mainstay of community nursing input. It can be rewarding to facilitate effective care that has a long-term impact on the health and well-being of patients. A typical example would be the patient with a venous leg ulcer progressing from holistic assessment identifying health needs and the causes of the ulcer through implementation of appropriate individualised planned care (e.g. compression therapy), to subsequent evaluation underpinned by education information and active encouragement in maintaining a healthier lifestyle to prevent recurrence (e.g. maintenance with compression hosiery), to eventual healing and discharge from the community nurse's caseload.

Keeping patients with a diagnosis of malignancy, particularly those receiving palliative treatment, active on my caseload allows the nursing team to develop relationships that form the basis of providing effective support to meet their needs. Planning significantly ahead ensures that the care provided will be of high quality anticipating need, and will therefore not simply be an emergency response which may fail due to resource constraints. The challenge of providing a fully coordinated package of care that enables a patient to choose to die in their home environment, which effectively supports relatives and significant others, can be one of the most challenging and rewarding elements of the District Nurse's role. The case history (see box) illustrates the coordination of an effective package of care.

Beyond visiting patients, planning, evaluating and coordinating packages of care, a significant portion of my time will be spent on other activities which focus more directly on the management and team element of the role. Weekly meetings are held with District Nurses from other bases and the clinical lead for the Primary Care Trust (PCT). This is to allow feedback from relevant strategic and PCT meetings and enables staff to cascade new initiatives, policies and

# Case history

As the District Nurse I was first made aware of Peter via a telephone referral from the oncology ward of the local hospital. Peter was 50 years old and had been diagnosed with a brain tumour, which was inoperable. He had been given a palliative course of radiotherapy as an in-patient. As a consequence his condition stabilised, and he was now ready for discharge into the community. The ward sister had contacted the District Nurse, as Peter had been given a poor prognosis and would require considerable support to maintain a good quality of life for him at home.

Initial dialogue with the sister of the oncology ward in advance of Peter's discharge was to establish and plan what help and equipment he would require. Peter needed help with most activities of living, as he was unstable on his feet, forgetful and prone to fitting. During the course of these conversations it became clear that more effective discharge planning could be achieved through meeting Peter and his family, and a case conference was arranged.

When preparing for a complex discharge, advance planning and a case conference can ensure that things go as smoothly a possible. Moreover this may prevent inappropriate readmission or delayed discharge of patients.

The case conference went very well – it enabled me to begin to develop a rapport not only with Peter but also with members of his family, who were keen to provide as much support and care as possible. It also enabled me to identify what possible equipment would be needed to facilitate discharge into the community. Peter was a tall, large man, factors not evident from telephone conversations. This knowledge enabled the correct size of hoist and slings to be ordered for him. Arrangements were made to facilitate discharge the following week subject to all equipment being in place, and further assessment of Peter's abilities would be left until this time, as his condition was changing from day to day.

Peter was subsequently discharged home. The timing of his discharge was coordinated and planned for an afternoon. I visited on the same afternoon to complete a holistic assessment of Peter's needs and ensure that his family were prepared for his first night at home. Peter contributed and was involved as much as possible in the assessment, although memory problems and poor concentration limited his abilities. Consequently, his wife provided much of the information. The nursing needs identified at this time were to provide psychological support for Peter and his wife; to monitor his symptoms, particularly headaches, and provide pain relief; to monitor the level and frequency of any fits; to provide catheter care; to monitor pressure areas; to meet identified hygiene needs; and to ensure that relatives and staff were safe and competent using the equipment provided. At this stage Peter was able to transfer safely from bed to chair with the assistance of one nurse or carer. Peter's family wished to provide all care in the evenings; therefore the initial package of care implemented was for nursing staff to visit in the morning and afternoon to provide care. Social services were not involved in providing care due to the unstable nature of his condition. Arrangements were made for the Macmillan Nurse to visit and his wife was informed of the availability of the Marie Curie Nursing Service, who would sit with Peter for several hours at a time, allowing her to leave Peter in safe hands.

Following the assessment I delegated his care to members of the nursing team. Two health care assistants visited each morning to assist with his hygiene needs, monitor pressure areas and provide catheter care. Their role included communication with other members of the team, particularly if there were changes in his condition or concerns raised by his family. Qualified staff visited in the afternoon again to meet his hygiene needs, but also to review the package of care and reassess his needs. I regularly reviewed his care as part of the team providing care. The GP and Macmillan Nurse also made regular visits to review Peter, with close liaison between all professionals involved. Peter's condition remained stable for several weeks, and during this time he enjoyed the company of his family and friends, positively benefiting from being able to contribute to family life. The nursing staff developed a good rapport with Peter and his wife and we were able to plan ahead for changes to his package of care as his needs and abilities altered. For example, issues in moving and handling and his eventual dependence on a hoist were carefully negotiated with him to meet not only his safety but that of the staff and his family.

Several weeks after discharge from hospital Peter had two major fits and his condition subsequently deteriorated. However, continual re-evaluation of his needs, monitoring of his condition and forward planning had allowed us to prepare for this and ensure that equipment such as syringe drivers and adequate pain relief were on hand. As he neared the terminal phase it became clear that although still very keen to help whenever possible, his family were finding it increasingly more distressing to assist in personal tasks. To ensure that adequate levels of care could be maintained his package of care was re-evaluated and was supported by input from the night nursing service and the hospice at home team.

Peter eventually died peacefully at home with all his family in attendance. On the day of his death the nursing teams provided all care to Peter and psychological support for his family. Members of the nursing

> team, at the request of his family, attended his funeral. On the subsequent bereavement visit his wife expressed heart-felt thanks to all the professionals who had been involved in Peter's care, saying that she felt the expertise, quality of care and coordination of all the professionals involved had surpassed her expectations in being able to achieve Peter's aim to die at home.

relevant documentation. This ensures that district nursing teams are working not in isolation but together to meet local and strategic developments and plans. Within this forum the District Nurses provide feedback from the various groups and working parties on which they may be representatives (for example benchmarking, guideline development, agenda for change, key skills framework), many of which will impact on future service delivery and standards.

## Other aspects of the role

Another essential element of my role is team management. It is important as a District Nurse that I remain aware of team dynamics and the strengths and weaknesses within the team, and relate this effectively to the needs of the local population. Working together to complete joint assessments and to observe the staff in practice enables me to identify the education and resources needed. Guiding staff in completing personal development plans linked to current key skills frameworks can enable me to encourage staff in the development of skills that will encourage personal development whilst also meeting the needs of the local community and the nursing team.

Nurse education and the inclusion of both pre- and post-registration students on placement in a primary care environment are essential. Due to the nature of one-to-one visits we would normally only have one pre-registration adult branch student on placement at any one time, although there may also be a post-registration student undertaking the degree pathway for a District Nurse qualification. The positive benefits of this are that the student experience is enriched by the personal commitment of time, communication and support that the mentor is able to give them.

My expectation of students on placement is that they will develop an understanding of community that encompasses the holistic concept of nursing practice. Aims fundamental to this would be the development and expansion of communication skills, both on a one-to-one basis with patients and from a wider perspective within the primary care team and across the multidisciplinary team, and utilisation of reflective skills to evaluate interventions and care plans, ultimately promoting the students' abilities to effectively link and utilise theoretical concepts to practice. The challenge for the District Nurse as a mentor is to ensure that the community environment actively encourages students to question practice and practitioners and enables them to reflect on what is done and what could be done (Canham and Moore, 2002).

## My role with students

As pre-registration students are usually in their third year, the expectation is that their level of skill and knowledge will be fairly well developed and that they will be able to utilise some of their previous experiences. Also, they are often a valuable resource for the district nursing team, providing up-to-date feedback from other health care environments. Students usually look forward to the latter part of the placement, as they are then able to take a small delegated caseload of patients and will experience first-hand autonomous practice. Although they often express anxiety at this time, this element of practice enables students to truly utilise their communication and reflective skills and facilitates the realisation of the placement aims. If my team are effective in supporting and mentoring students that pass through the community environment, the knowledge and skills that each student develops on this placement will reflect positively not only on their subsequent education but also their future practice.

The most rewarding element of this branch of nursing and the primary motivator in my post as a District Nurse is that the role of community practitioner truly encompasses the holistic philosophy underpinning nursing practice. Inextricably linked to this is an ability to work as an autonomous and reflective practitioner making decisions based on sound evidence-based practice. Care is planned, implemented and evaluated in complete negotiation with clients, and all aspects of life and the community in which they live are taken into consideration. However, the challenge will always be to provide optimum care within available resources (Roberts, 1996). I feel it is important to function as the patient's advocate, creating an open and supportive atmosphere that is supportive of patient choice and decisions, a philosophy echoed by current government policy (Department of Health, 2001, 2003, 2004b) that demands 'patient focused' health care.

## The developing role of the District Nurse

The management of complex care packages and being able to effectively coordinate a range of services to meet a clients needs and improve the quality of an individual patient's experience of ill health can be justifiably satisfying, although the challenges of resource limitation and ineffective methods of communication which delay the implementation of packages, particularly when planning complex hospital discharges, can be disappointing. I find it particularly frustrating to achieve effective communication across a range of services, especially when this is compounded not only by the physical barriers of differing locations but also sadly by the narrow focus of different professional perspectives and the desire to protect professional territory. These difficulties and the spectre of cost effectiveness inevitably affect the quality of care provided.

My role as a District Nurse, along with community nursing, has changed considerably in recent years, and this looks set to continue to evolve. There are and will be increasing numbers of elderly patients with acute and chronic conditions nursed at home with fewer families to care for them (Robinson, 2002). In addition, earlier hospital discharge and increasingly complex procedures are occurring in the community. The shift in focus of health care policy from secondary to primary care has inevitably led to an increase in the demands placed on the District Nurse. As a District Nurse I am frequently caught between meeting the needs of the client and maintaining standards and quality within the inevitable staff shortages and resource limitations. These challenges are particularly evident in the inner city environment, with its inherent problems of social deprivation and health inequality, where my caseload is located.

Changes to the structure of community health care provision, such as intermediate care (e.g. hospital at home, rapid assessment teams), have been created to address these issues, although they can be viewed conflictingly as both supporting and eroding the role of the District Nurse. Future trends identified in NHS reform and government legislation to promote the public health agenda and the inception of community matrons highlight the importance of effectively managing long-term conditions (Department of Health, 2000, 2001, 2004a, 2005a,b). I feel that the District Nurse holds a uniquely significant position for meeting the Government's agenda. Skills in health promotion and the coordination of complex care pathways will put District Nurses in a prime position to promote and take forward inter-professional initiatives, promote collaborative working and remain at the forefront of primary care in the future.

## Editor's comments

It is often difficult on a short placement for a student nurse to appreciate the breadth of responsibility that the District Nurse has. Helen as team leader has overall responsibility for the assessment, planning and overview of about 200 patients. She is responsible for her staff and students that are on placement. She has to manage this team by delegation and inspiration. How does this role differ from that of the ward sister in a hospital? There are a number of similarities, but also there are key differences. The ward sister or senior nurse is physically accessible – if the junior nurse or health care assistant has a clinical problem, then the sister is usually only a matter of metres away. The district nursing sister does not have this luxury. She must assess the needs of all new patients and make sure that she allocates that care to appropriately experienced staff. She needs to support her staff from a distance. How do you think you would work as a staff nurse in that sort of team? Many students believe that they require several years of hospital experience before they venture into the community. Whilst there are a number of advantages in gaining some hospital experience before working in the community, a number of newly qualified staff enter directly into community work. Often these are confident people who have worked as health care assistants before training as a nurse, but this is not always the case. Provided you get a job in a team that will provide you with a good preceptorship programme, you will soon develop the skills and confidence required of a community nurse. The privilege of being invited into someone's home and building up a relationship with them and their family is one that gives tremendous job satisfaction.

# References

Barr, J. (2001) Effective communication in primary care. In: *Nursing in Primary Care: A Handbook for Students* (eds. N. Watson and C. Wilkinson). Palgrave, Basingstoke.

Canham, J. (2002) Setting the scene: concepts of specialist practitioner and specialist mentor. In: *Mentorship in Community: Nursing Challenges & Opportunities* (eds. J. Canham and J. Bennett). Blackwell Science, Oxford.

Canham, J. and Moore, S. (2002) Learning approaches in the practice context. In: *Mentorship in Community Nursing: Challenges & Opportunities* (eds. J. Canham and J. Bennett). Blackwell Science, Oxford.

Department of Health (2000) *The NHS Plan*. HMSO, London.

Department of Health (2001) *The National Service Framework for Older People*. HMSO, London.

Department of Health (2003) *Standards for Better Health*. HMSO, London.

Department of Health (2004a) *The NHS Improvement Plan*. HMSO, London.

Department of Health (2004b) *Choosing Health – Making Healthier Choices Easier*. HMSO, London.

Department of Health (2005a) *The National Service Framework for Long Term Conditions*. HMSO, London.

Department of Health (2005b) *Supporting People with Long Term Conditions. Liberating the Talents of Nurses Who Care for People with Long Term Conditions*. HMSO, London.

Roberts, B. (1996) Health at home. In: *Community Health Care Nursing Principles for Practice* (eds. S. Twinn, B. Roberts and S. Andrews). Butterworth-Heinemann, Oxford.

Robinson, A. (2002) District nursing. In: *Mentorship in Community Nursing: Challenges & Opportunities* (eds. J. Canham and J. Bennett). Blackwell Science, Oxford.

UKCC (1994) *The Future of Professional Practice: the Council's Standards for Education and Practice Following Registration*. UKCC, London.

# CHAPTER 4

# The experience of a community health care assistant

*Ann Clements*

## Editor's introduction

If you have just read Chapter 3, written by Helen the district nursing sister, you will realise that district nursing requires a team approach led by the sister/charge nurse. Within that team are the qualified staff nurse and the health care assistant (HCA). Ann is a health care assistant who has been working in the community for many years. Prior to working in the community she was a health care assistant in a hospital setting, and she saw her move into the community as a way of developing her career. The role of the HCA in the community can be quite different from that in the hospital, as community HCAs must be trained to undertake specific tasks in patients' homes without the direct supervision of the qualified nurse. Therefore they must be able to work in an independent way, but always be aware of their limitations. The district nursing sister will carry out the initial patient assessment and then delegate subsequent care to either a qualified nurse or the HCA. You can begin to see the importance of teamwork, multi-skilling, delegation and good communication.

As you read through Ann's account you will see what an interesting and responsible role she has within the team. If you have any opportunities to accompany some HCAs when on your community experience, make sure you work with as many as you can. Most community HCAs have a wealth of experience and you can learn a tremendous amount about managing care, building up relationships with a variety of patients and what it is like to work in the community team. The other important aspect that you can learn from the community HCA relates to the fact that many of the people that work as HCAs are from the very local population. Thus they know the area well, with all its problems, facilities and opportunities. Many of the qualified nurses that you will work with have not been brought up in the local community and often live some miles away, so use your placement with the community HCA to teach you about the local community and its health and social care needs.

Reflect upon Ann's role, the way that her skills and training are used, her responsibilities, her place in the team, and her relationships with her patients. How do you think her skills will compare to yours when you qualify?

# The community health care assistant

## My background

I first came into this profession many years ago, more for convenience than anything else. I had two small children and wanted to go out to work, but did not want to leave the children with strangers. I saw an advertisement for a part-time nursing auxiliary for two nights a week working in a hospital environment, on an orthopaedic ward. No experience was required, as training would be given. It required good communication skills and a caring nature, which I felt that I had. I also felt that being a mother and managing a household would be an advantage. I applied and was very pleased and a little surprised when I was offered the job. I enjoyed this work very much, soon realising that although I had first come into the job for convenience, I enjoyed the work: caring for others, communicating with all different types of people, and the feeling that by one small thing, whether it be helping an old lady with her teeth or giving the gent round the corner a shave, it made individuals feel better. After a number of years working in the hospital I felt I wanted more of a challenge. My children were grown up and reasonably independent. I saw an advert for a job working in the community as a nursing auxiliary, or health care assistant as we are now called. Again I felt that I had the life skills and the experience for this role, so I applied and was offered the job.

# My skills

I do feel that my years working within the hospital helped me to prepare for my role within the community. As with the hospital job, no formal qualifications were required, but I do feel that working in the community would have been very daunting if this had been my first role. I think the essential skills required for this role are good communication skills. Being able to communicate with a variety of different people at all levels is very important. For instance, each day I will be looking after approximately six to eight different patients, many of whom have concerned relatives. I will also need to communicate with my district nursing sister and other staff within my team, and occasionally I will have to telephone a GP to report back on a patient's condition. Being able to work on one's own is also important, as within the community setting you very much work alone, but you have always the backup of your fellow staff members and other networks. The qualified nurses will assess the patient's needs initially and then plan the care which I have to follow. The care plans can be either written or verbal.

My role as an HCA is not an easy one, I have to act upon the instructions and guidance of the qualified nurses, but at the same time I am in the patient's house on my own and if I feel that the patient's condition has changed from when the qualified nurse initially assessed them, then I have to have the confidence to say to the qualified nurse, 'I think Mr Smith might benefit from a different form of action'.

# My role

I would summarise my role as one which supports the qualified staff within the community nursing team. This involves giving nursing care to individuals who live in their own homes. My responsibilities are to the GPs, members of staff within my practice and (primarily) the individual patients within my care. I also have a responsibility to follow all health and safety regulations as decided by the Primary Care Trust.

My typical week starts on a Monday morning. I work 18.75 hours per week, covering Monday to Friday mornings. All staff within the team meet in the office of the health centre where we are based at. Each member of staff has what is called a 'planner': this is a form listing all patients in our care, their addresses, treatment required and the days that visits are required. I go over my planner and transfer individual names and details to a diary sheet, which is a form detailing visits, day, date and name of staff member. This then becomes the list of my duties for that morning. All this planning takes about 30 minutes, after which I leave the health centre and start my visits. This time in the office gives staff members time to discuss any queries or concerns about patients and to take any new patients that have been referred. Also, some patients may require two staff to visit them; if so, then it is at this stage of the day that this needs to be organised, with a time being agreed for when we are going to meet up.

## My journey starts

After listing my patients for that morning I then decide on what route I will take. This is not as obvious as it might sound, as I have to take into account the patients' individual needs; the time at which I have arranged to meet up with another member of staff; what the shortest route is; and which route avoids the busiest traffic. I leave the health centre and start my visits for that morning. I can have anything from four to eight patients per shift, depending on what kind of visit is required and how many staff are available to cover all the patients. I travel in my car to visit each patient: this can be in their own home, or they might be living with a relative or even in a residential home. When I arrive I introduce myself, explaining who I am and what I have come to do. I carry an identification badge with my photo and name on which can be shown at any time when asked for.

## The patient's home

Each patient will have their own nursing notes with them in the house. These contain all the relevant information about the individual that I or other community staff will need. This includes the care plan, which explains the problem and what nursing care is required. I always read these notes before starting any procedure, even if I know the patient quite well, as there may have been a change in circumstances or condition since the last time I visited this patient. After reading the care plan and identifying the relevant treatment required, I then prepare the materials, equipment and area to carry out this procedure safely and effectively. Having discussed what I need to do with the patient, I carry out the procedure. Following that I need to return all materials and equipment to safe storage and leave the room as it was before. I need to record in the patient's nursing notes all activities carried out and any concerns or complications with the procedure, signing and dating it appropriately. There is rarely time for social conversation with the patients, but I try very hard to make a few minutes, either before, during or after the procedure, to talk to them about their family or how they are coping generally. Often I am the only person that they see that day, and sometimes the only person they see that week.


## Survival skills


I have found that having a good sense of humour and being broad-minded are great advantages, as people are very different in their own environment. Most people when in a hospital setting are quite insecure and sometimes frightened. However, people in their own homes are far more confident and you see their true personality. I once visited a gentleman who was in his 80s. We got chatting and he asked me how many children I had. Not thinking that he was doing anything other than making conversation, I explained that I had two children. He immediately asked, with a big toothless grin on his face, 'Would you like another?'! I do not know who laughed the most: me or his wife. Then there was the time when one of my calls was to a man for a leg dressing. After my introduction and explanation of why I was visiting, I asked to see his nursing notes. When I turned round he had his hands under the covers of the bed and brought out an artificial leg, saying 'Some of the other nurses find it easier to put it on the table by the window to do the dressing'. He had such a serious expression on his face. For a split second I was unsure how to react: was he joking or did he have some sort of psychological problem? However, he saw my dilemma and started laughing and said, 'You're the fourth one I've got with that one'.

I finish my shift at lunchtime. Each day has a similar pattern, but no two days are the same, as I visit different patients on different days. Some patients only need weekly visits, while others might need three visits a week – it all depends upon the individual patient's needs. I can travel approximately 60–100 miles a week going from one patient to another, but this can vary depending the area you cover. I work in a city centre, so the mileage is quite low compared with community staff that work in rural areas. The greatest frustration of working in the city is the difficulty in parking close to the patient's house.

Here are some of the typical patients I visit within my role as a HCA. Some patients require general nursing care, and often these are people who are in the last stages of their life. Depending on the individual patient's needs, either one or two staff will visit. Often two are required to assist with the moving and handling of the patient, as the last thing you want to do is to pull a patient about who is already in a great deal of pain or discomfort. We will give them a full bed bath, change their night wear, empty catheter bags or change incontinence pads, change the bed when necessary, check pressure areas and leave them in a safe and comfortable position. We also give reassurance and comfort to carers and family members as appropriate.

I have patients with deep wounds that require packing and dressing to allow them to drain and heal from the bottom up. Another large part of my caseload is patients who have leg ulcers; these can have many different forms of dressing applied, depending on the ulcer and the best dressing to promote effective healing for that individual. In addition, there are the simple dressings; these could be from surgery or cuts and falls. Some patients require blood pressure monitoring on a weekly, fortnightly or monthly basis, depending on their condition and instructions from the GP, and venous blood samples need to be taken as requested by either the hospital or the GP, often for patients who would be unable to get to the GP surgery or out-patient department. Eye drops must be administered as prescribed by the hospital or the GP for patients that do not have the physical ability or coordination to administer their own. All of these examples form part of my routine work. Each patient will have been delegated to me by the district nursing sister to carry out the care according to the care plan.

All patients are seen by the district nursing sister, who will carry out a holistic assessment on that individual to meet their needs and to refer on to other services if needed. If any nursing needs are identified the district nursing sister will complete a set of nursing notes specific to that individual. All relevant information will be recorded in these notes and a care plan will be drawn up. This will show the illness or condition requiring treatment, the expectations and the plan of care, i.e. how many times visits are required, what treatment or medication is prescribed and how to carry out treatment. It is important for any changes to be recorded in the notes and reported back to the District Nurse or qualified nurse so that action can be taken to rectify any changes or complications.

The student nurses on placement in the community spend most of their time with the qualified nurses. Most of the students are in their second or third year of training and normally spend 12 weeks on their placement. They only come out with me once or twice, to see what the role of the nursing auxiliary is.

## My ongoing training and development

There are lots of in-house training courses (e.g. health and safety, basic life support, safe handling and moving, fire prevention, infection control) to attend, which are very important for this role. Most of these courses are mandatory and everyone must attend. Another qualification relevant to this role is NVQ Level 3 in care; this is not mandatory, but desirable. In addition there are discussions and informal training that I receive from the experienced and qualified staff within the team.

# My job satisfaction

What I enjoy most about my role is meeting so many different people: little old ladies with their blue rinses; cantankerous old men (and women); poorly terminal patients; and the patients we maybe only see for two to three weeks. The most important thing is that these individuals want to be in their own homes, and this service provides the care to enable their wishes to be carried out. I enjoy the different roles of this job, from a simple blood pressure reading to a more complicated visit, which might involve visiting a dying patient with a member of the qualified staff. I have met many different people over the years and made many good friends by way of other staff members and the patients and families that I have met through my role as a health care assistant. When I visit a patient who is terminally ill and continue those visits for a number of months, I cannot help but get to know them and their families personally. I also cannot help feeling a sense of loss when this patient dies, but I still to this day feel a sense of achievement that I helped, be it in only a small way, the final wishes of this patient and their family to be carried out, and for this patient to end their days in their own home with dignity and quality, and most of all surrounded by their families.

It has been important to be able to change and move with the growing need of the service. My role has changed greatly since I first started. When I first started my role was basically to help to get patients up in the morning, give them either a strip wash or a bath/shower, help them to dress, and leave them safely for the day. Now my role is nothing like that. The only wash or bed bath I give now is to terminally ill patients, as for other patients this is designated as social care and is not part of the community nurse's role. My duties include simple wound dressings, blood pressure monitoring, blood sugar monitoring, catheter care or collecting samples (e.g. venous blood or urine). It has been a great challenge to move with the service, but a very enjoyable and rewarding one. The difficulties I feel are that HCAs know their limitations and do not step over the line of their training or abilities, and they need to know where the boundary between the HCA and the qualified nurse's role lies. This is a very real concern, as more and more roles have been given to the nursing auxiliary and knowing where our areas of responsibility lie is not easy – the boundaries seem to be forever changing. As the role has expanded, so has my confidence, but the difficulty is in saying 'no' when feeling pressurised into taking on new roles that I feel unprepared for.

The role of the HCA can go one or two ways. I feel that it has reached its maximum at this time. However, the development of a regulated, well-structured training plan with recognised guidelines seems to be a real possibility. I feel that there could be a recognised qualification for nursing auxiliaries, not to the standard of the qualified nurse, but by a registration for nursing auxiliaries who have achieved a recognised standard and quality, as set out by the nursing standards. The other way would be for nothing to change and for nursing auxiliaries to stay as they are, but there is then the problem of where and when do we stop and at what point do we say no.

## Editor's comments

Somewhat sadly, the student's placement in the community usually only involves a short placement with the health care assistant. As Ann says, this normally lasts for just one or two shifts so that you can appreciate the role that they play in the team. This is due to the nursing and midwifery training regulations, which specify that students need to be mentored by a qualified nurse. Whilst this is understandable, in that students need to be mentored by experienced and qualified professionals, it belittles the skills and work that people like Ann have and do. People like Ann have a tremendous amount of experience and skill that is of tremendous value to the student nurse. They may not have the refined skills of teaching and mentoring that qualified nurses have and thus as a student you may have to take the lead in learning from people like Ann. This means active observation, asking non-threatening questions, reflecting upon their practice and generally being an enthusiastic student.

What have you learnt from reading Ann's account? She demonstrates the importance of assessment, delegation, communication, teamwork, organisation and planning. Ann also demonstrates the importance of personal skills, such as the ability to relate to a variety of patients with very different conditions. Whether your first job as a qualified nurse is in the community or in a hospital you will almost certainly be working in a team that has HCAs as key members. As you read Ann's account you will obviously be very impressed with her dedication and commitment to her job. But Ann is not the unusual exception: the majority of HCAs are equally committed and skilled, and with the right leadership, training, support and job descriptions they form a key part of the nursing team.

# CHAPTER 5

# The experiences of a District Nurse and practice educator

*Ruth Rojhan*

## Editor's introduction

Ruth's account is that of an experienced District Nurse who has an 80% patient caseload and a 20% educational input. If you were to work in the community and then decide to undertake the degree in community nursing to become a district nursing sister, then you would be allocated to someone like Ruth who would be your practice-based teacher/mentor. To practice as a health visitor or District Nurse requires a post-registration qualification in Community Nursing, usually at degree level, although some are at Masters level. This degree is also becoming more frequently seen as a prerequisite for other roles within the community, particularly when that role involves specialist practice or leading a team. Thus practice nurses and school nurses are increasingly being encouraged and supported to undertake such studies.

For 80% of her time Ruth works in direct patient care and leads a team of community nurses. In this way her role is very similar to that of Helen, the district nursing sister in Chapter 3, and you should compare the two accounts. One significant difference it that Helen works in the middle of a large inner city catchment area, whereas Ruth works in a more rural county and spends a considerable amount of time travelling from one patient to another.

A great similarity that comes out from both Helen's and Ruth's accounts is the way that they talk about their patients as people that they know and like and how they go to visit them in their homes (not houses!). A second significant similarity is the feeling that they both work in teams whose members are friends, and it is noticeable that students entering these teams become part of what almost seems to be a family (see Stuart's and Sarah's student nurse accounts in Chapters 2 and 12). Whilst this closeness of relationships can be very supportive and pleasant, there are some potential disadvantages and not everyone feels comfortable with closeness, preferring more distant relationships. This may be what attracts some people to the community work: it certainly has a peculiar combination of working independently, yet within a strong family-like team atmosphere. There are certainly some similarities between family life and community nursing. In my family we tend to start the day together with a somewhat rushed breakfast which is combined with preparing to go out to our various jobs/schools/colleges. We then depart, often having minimal conversation with each other, which if it does occur usually involves very practical points such as 'Bring some food in for tea' or 'Don't forget to phone the plumber to arrange repairs'. Likewise, with the community team, the start of the day is a rushed coffee in the same office during which essential business details are sorted out prior to everyone rushing off to their busy schedule for that day. Both the family and the community team usually return at the end of the day. Most are quite tired; some are quite elated that they had a good day and everything went really well; others are frustrated because the opposite happened; some return wanting to talk; and others prefer a bit of quiet.

This family picture is an interesting analogy of community working and one that can be taken further. For instance, is the person who lives alone a bit like the specialist nurse? Is the mother figure the team leader? Is one of the family very hardworking and can always be relied upon, while another is more laid back? Are some very tidy and good at paperwork whilst others are just messy and disorganised? I have four children in my family. As a family we generally get on quite well together, but rarely does a day go by without some form of argument or door slamming! But we are a strong family. I think community teams are like this – it's not a place of perfect harmony and perfect communication, but it is a place of commitment to each other with a common corporate aim yet strong individual function.

Ruth's account is full of the realities of community nursing, from the closeness of the bond between a longstanding patient to the traumas of being bitten by the pet rabbit. Ruth's specialist input into community nursing is her role as a practice educator, and this combination of roles allows her to teach and supervise the future District Nurses, hopefully avoiding the theory–practice gap.

# A District Nurse and practice educator

## My role

I work as a District Nurse (DN) with a responsibility for the education and training of community nurses. This was formerly called a community practice teacher (CPT) in district nursing. The CPT role has been superseded in many areas by that of a lead mentor, although mentorship does not cover the full responsibilities of my role as a lead professional practice educator for my Primary Care Trust.

I have an interesting and challenging role in which I am responsible for:

- A clinical caseload which consists of a range of patients attached to a GP practice
- Management of the community nursing team attached to that caseload
- Practice education and in-service training for the Primary Care Trust as part of a team of three CPTs
- Education and training of pre-registration student nurses who spend placement time with the community nursing teams
- Education and training of student District Nurses undertaking the post-registration BSc in Community Health Nurse (District Nursing)

## My typical week

I work Monday to Friday from 8:30 a.m. until 5:00 p.m., which, after working shifts and weekends for most of my previous nursing career, came as a great luxury, and although this meant a reduction in salary due to the loss of the shift allowance, it allows me to organise my personal life to a greater degree and juggle the family/work balance (Tausig and Fenwick, 2001). In theory I spend my time in an 80/20 split, with 80% of my time in clinical practice working with patients and 20% of the time undertaking the educative part of my role as one of a team of three within the Trust. In reality this does not always work out this precisely, depending on the pressures and priorities which occur, with clinical emergencies taking priority over my educational responsibilities.

I work in a county PCT and my patients can be from any setting in the locality, and this is one of the aspects of my job which makes it so interesting. I have nursed patients who lived in a variety of environments, including houses, flats and residential homes, farms and caravans, over shops and pubs, and even in probation hostels. This diversity enhances the individuality of patient care and increases my job satisfaction, an aspect shared by many people who work in the community.

Visiting my patients takes up a lot of my time, and in part that is because, in rural areas particularly, travelling to the patients can be time-consuming and can mean that I see patients with very complex and wide-ranging problems, which is again a common feature of community nursing (Lauder *et al.*, 2001). Urban visits also have their drawbacks, such as roads with double yellow lines and one-way streets, which can make parking and navigating difficult. District nurse are not exempt from receiving parking tickets unfortunately! Some of my patients are able to come to see me at the health centre where I am based, and in order to facilitate this I also run a variety of clinics, which include care of post-operative and traumatic wounds, leg ulcers, and continence. This allows the patients to have greater control over how they plan their day, rather than waiting in for me to visit, especially if they are at work or have other commitments. It also enables me to see more patients in the time allowed, although not seeing them at home can limit the aspects of patient individuality which I previously referred to as being one of the rewarding features in the job.

In my role of nurse educator, I plan and spend time with pre-registration nursing students in order to facilitate their learning about community nursing. In this, I have a responsibility to ensure that the student has the potential learning experience to appreciate the extent and variety of district nursing in order to understand the width and breadth that the term community can encompass (Meegan and Mitchell, 2001). Student nurses spend a placement of 16 weeks with the team, which gives them many opportunities to explore the varied complexities encompassed in the district nursing role.

The post-registration district nursing students have an entirely different experience. They are already qualified, and generally experienced nurses and are undertaking a post-registration degree specialising in district nursing. Their course, which spans 48 weeks, is divided equally between learning in the university setting and learning in the community setting. As a general rule, one district nursing student will be allocated to me as a practice educator for all of their 48 week course. Some days are spent at the university, undertaking theory components of the course, and others are spent in the community, undertaking set experiences and a supervised caseload. The student will shadow the CPT in order to learn about community nursing, and at the end of the course must be able to take on the work and role of a District Nurse. This entails a much more detailed programme of training, and my role is to support the student in this, as well as acting as a role model.

The other aspect of my educative role is that of training and supervision of members of the community nursing team in order that they remain up to date and effective in their work. This not only consists of assisting with the provision of the mandatory training set out by the Primary Care Trust, but also ensuring that current practice is evidence-based and takes into account new policy directives from the Department of Health. This means that I must find time in my week to read nursing journals and access professional forums to make certain that I remain up to date myself.

## Patient care

The typical District Nurse caseload is difficult to describe, as it is largely dependant on the population that it serves, which can be very diverse. The make-up of the local population will be reflected quite clearly in the identified health needs. Significant factors are: the percentage of older people; average levels of income and deprivation; cultural make-up; and attitudes to smoking/alcohol etc. All of these factors will have an impact on health needs and the resulting caseload of the District Nurse. The District Nurse must profile the demography and epidemiology of the local population and maximise its application in order to ensure that care is targeted appropriately and cost-effectively (Worth, 2001). Patient category and frequency of visiting have a major influence on the workload. Patients on the caseload require input at varying intervals, depending on the reason for nursing input, the complexity of the care required, any complicating factors, and patient concordance and individual needs.

Despite the variety of nursing care that a District Nurse may undertake, a common nursing practice for nearly all District Nurses is that of treating patients who have leg ulcers, which involves the assessment of causation by the use of a Doppler tool, as well as the application of appropriate compression bandaging (Meyer *et al.*, 2002). In the UK, leg ulcer treatment accounts for 1.3% of the total health care budget and up to 90% are treated in the community. It is vital that patients with a leg ulcer have a full holistic assessment as lack of this may lead to costly and inappropriate treatment. For example, applying compression bandaging compression to a limb where arterial supply is compromised may result in gangrene, whereas withholding compression where there is venous insufficiency may lead to failure to heal and deterioration of the ulcer (Hofman, 2000). Assessment may also include description of the wound, sometimes by using photography. This has implications for patient confidentiality, especially if the photography session takes place in the patient's own home, and care must be taken not to include household objects which identify the patient. Caring for a patient's wound must also include a negotiated agreement with the patient, as the District Nurse relies on the patient's concordance with treatment whilst not being monitored 24 hours of the day (Taylor, 2002). This puts the onus on the patient being a partner in the care, as well as being confident in contacting the District Nurse in the event of possible deterioration between visits. It is important that the nurse ensures that equipment and dressing stocks are maintained in the patient's home too, as it is not possible to pop into the treatment room as if it were a hospital ward. All dressings are obtained on patient prescription, and recently nurse prescribing has made an impact on the ease of obtaining dressings for District Nurses (Latter and Courtenay, 2004). On average, leg ulcers will take up to 12 weeks to heal with compression therapy, and some may take up to 9 months, so patients become accustomed to the nursing team visiting them and this helps to build therapeutic relationships. As well as the dressing treatment, care will also include health promotion to inform patients about caring for their legs to facilitate a good circulation and an adequate diet to encourage effective wound healing.

Opportunistic health promotion takes place as an ongoing activity during the visits, and the District Nurse is in a prime position to reinforce maintenance of healthy lifestyles, including smoking cessation and exercise.

## How I got into this job: experience and qualities required

My current role consists of holding a clinical caseload. I initially started work as a community staff nurse and then qualified as a District Nurse, and this gave me the experience which enabled me to take on this additional practice education role.

The current District Nurse is required to study for an average of 48 weeks to obtain the BSc Community Health Nurse (D.N.) Specialist practitioner qualification. This is a post-registration course undertaken in a university and may also include the nurse prescribing qualification. The course is often run jointly with health visitor students as part of inter-professional education because both jobs share similar values and knowledge. Then I undertook the Community Practice Teacher Diploma, a two-year part-time course which prepared me for the educative side of my job by introducing me to the theories and application of teaching and learning.

My earliest experience of district nursing was going out with my mother, who was also a District Nurse. During school holidays I would sit in the car whilst she did her visits, and was occasionally invited in by patients. Although I could not be present whilst care was being given, I was able to see how meeting patients and communicating with them in their own environment gave richness to the nurse–patient relationship, which I feel is more difficult to appreciate in a hospital setting (Williams, 2001). As a District Nurse, it is possible to learn lots from patients, not only about how they manage their disease, but also how they relate to their world. I learnt to crochet from one of my mother's patients, a skill I still have to this day. The District Nurse, whilst remaining a guest in the patient's home (Taylor, 2002), also becomes part of the family and a friend. However, sometimes this makes discharging patients a difficult or painful undertaking. One of the skills I have had to learn when becoming a District Nurse myself is that of terminating the relationship when the programme of care is complete. Although there is much written about best practice for discharging patients from hospital (McKenna *et al.*, 2000), there is little to direct District Nurses in this area, and most acquire this skill on the job through experiential learning.

Another important characteristic which District Nurses need to have is an interest in patients as individuals, and being able to negotiate without being judgemental. For instance, I have visited patients in a variety of settings and have encountered all sorts of pets, from the normal cats and dogs to a monkey, snakes and other exotica. Attempting to undertake a sterile dressing whilst the pet rabbit is hopping around the room can be fraught with danger, as attempting to stroke one resulted in a trip to Accident and Emergency for a tetanus injection following a bite! Negotiating care within the patient's home must also take into account the professional responsibilities that the nurse has in relation to Health and Safety at Work Act 1974. During my work I have learned the necessity of negotiating with patients in order to work safely in the home environment and to take into account patient choice. When undertaking palliative care for terminally ill patients the District Nurse must be sensitive to many normally private issues. For example, many married couples are still sleeping together in a double bed, and may have been married for many years. To ask them to sleep apart, so that the patient can be nursed safely in a hospital bed, can be insensitive at such a time, and can be detrimental to the grieving process as well as the nurse–patient relationship. However, the District Nurse must be mindful of her obligations under the Code of Conduct (Nursing and Midwifery Council, 2004) and resolve these issues with care and consideration to both patients, family and care staff.

## Pleasures, challenges and future directions

The importance of the clinical experience and a need for high-quality practice placements emphasises the responsibilities that CPTs have within community nurse education. I hold a recordable teaching qualification considered by many to be more exacting than that required of their hospital counterparts, and for this I have been rewarded both financially and with higher status than my District Nurse colleagues. However, there have been longstanding concerns regarding the lack of standards of community practice teachers (Hudson, 2000). Keeping myself up to date and working utilising evidence-based practice requires self-discipline in order to maintain the necessary high standards expected of me as a role model and educator. Much of my work is done in isolation, with few peers for support. Indeed, this is the nature of district nursing. Working in partnership with universities is the rhetoric, but in reality there is still a practice–theory gap evident within the relationships between clinical educators and university lecturers. However, over the years I have seen many students successfully through their courses in both pre- and post-registration training, and certainly that brings its own rewards. Working relationships with students over long months of study have forged longstanding friendships which have enriched my working life, and have also resulted in my being able to tap into a network of qualified nurses and the knowledge base that they hold.

The memories of patients and their families are another aspect of district nursing which provides much pleasure, especially those where I feel I have been able to make a difference to their lives, as is the case for many nurses. There are also those who I might prefer to forget, which is true of all aspects of nursing. There are patients who have been particularly challenging and really test the skills of the District Nurse. These are usually those whose condition is complex or unusual, or whose response to coping with their illness is different from the norm.

There are also challenging students, who for a number of reasons have not felt the enthusiasm for community nursing, and I hoped to inspire these people, although that is not always possible.

For the future, traditional models of higher education are now being challenged and new models that concentrate on evidencing the development of knowledge through practice are emerging. The move from the classroom to the practice is set to continue. The future of practice-based education in new and innovative ways seems secure. The transition towards different ways of learning in higher education has led to a need for new strategies for facilitating and assessing within practice. This is the test and challenge for the future practice educators.

> With a strong educational knowledge base to draw on and currency within the clinical field, the practice educator within specialist practice will have the opportunity to develop a structured educational support in partnership with higher education and mentors and implement more innovative ways for students to work and learn and collect evidence for verification of learning outcomes. (Stevens, 2003. p. 31)

## Students on placement

During a placement in the community, students will become familiar with the local facilities and how the population interacts within their neighbourhood.

Each community is distinct and individual, with its own special needs and priorities. Gaining an appreciation of this is one of the most important aspects of the student experience. To this end, students are encouraged to go out and explore the local environment and gain empathy and insight into what it is like to live in that particular place. This necessitates a degree of motivation and enthusiasm as well as initiative on the part of students in order that they take advantage of the diversity of experience which is on offer.

It is impossible for students to cover every type of ill-health condition as the scope is so wide-ranging, but to benefit most from the learning experience, it is useful to take the opportunity to select two or three conditions which interest them the most and study them in depth, with reference to the application of theory to practice.

Students will be expected to work as part of a team and gain a working knowledge of collaborative, multi-agency working practices, and hopefully this will facilitate a sense of fulfilment and achievement by the end of the placement.

District Nurse caseloads are under increasing pressure due to the increasing elderly population and shift to community care, resulting in earlier hospital discharge. These aspects of care are increasing and have become more complex and time-consuming in nature. *Our Health, Our Care, Our Say: a New Direction for Community Services* (Department of Health, 2006) contains some welcome opportunities for improving community services, and recognises that community nurses play a key part in leading those improvements.

## Editor's comments

I am sure you will agree that Ruth has an interesting and fulfilling role as both clinician and teacher. What differences did you see in the way that she carried out her role and the way in which Helen carried out her similar role? It is interesting to note the changes in the district nursing role over recent years and how this trend appears to be increasing. This is due partly to the increasing age of our population and the chronic illnesses that accompany increasing age. It is also due to the increasing use of technology and advances in medical science that allow patients to be treated in hospital in different ways and discharged into the community under the care of skilled practitioners. There are exciting and challenging times ahead for community nurses – do you think you would enjoy working in the community once you have qualified?

Have you reflected upon the analogy of the community team as a family? If so, has this helped you appreciate the different roles and forms of communication that seem to be occurring in your community placement. If you were to describe your community placement in terms of a family, what would that family be like? Would it be *The Simpsons*, *Malcolm in the Middle* or *The Royle Family*? If you are still on your community placement, then share this idea of the community team as a family and ask different members of the team how they would describe their perception of their community family – the results will be very interesting, just as interesting as if you do the same exercise with your own family. Try it and see.

# References

Department of Health (2006) *Our Health, Our Care, Our Say: A New Direction for Community Services*. HMSO, London.

Hofman, D. (2000) Management of leg ulcers. *Nursing Standard*, **14**(29) Quick Reference Guide 15.

Hudson, R. (2000) *Professional Briefing. Practice Educators. Preparing for New Roles in the NHS*. CPHVA, London.

Latter, S. and Courtenay, M. (2004) Effectiveness of nurse prescribing: a review of the literature. *Journal of Clinical Nursing*, **13**(1), 26–32.

Lauder, W., Reynolds, W., Reilly, V. and Angus, N. (2001) The role of district nurses in caring for people with mental health problems who live in rural settings. *Journal of Clinical Nursing*, **10**, 337–44.

McKenna, H., Keeney, S., Glenn, A. and Gordon, P. (2000) Discharge planning: an exploratory study. *Journal of Clinical Nursing*, **9**(4), 594–601.

Meegan, R. and Mitchell, A. (2001) It's not community round here, it's neigh-bourhood: neighbourhood change and cohesion in urban regeneration poli-cies. *Urban Studies*, **38**(12), 2167–94.

Meyer, F. J., Burnand, K. G., Lagattolla, N. R. F. and Eastham, D. (2002) Ran-domized clinical trial comparing the efficacy of two bandaging regimens in the treatment of venous leg ulcers. *British Journal of Surgery*, **89**(1), 40–4.

Nursing and Midwifery Council (2004) *The Code of Professional Conduct: Standards for Conduct, Performance and Ethics*. Nursing and Midwifery Council, London.

Stevens, D. (2003) The practice educator in specialist community practice. *Journal of Community Nursing*, **17**(2), 30–1.

Tausig, M. and Fenwick, R. (2001) Unbinding time: alternate work schedules and work-life balance. *Journal of Family and Economic Issues*, **22**(2), 101–19.

Taylor, B. (2002) Nurse: patient partnership: rhetoric or reality? *Journal of Community Nursing*, **16**(3), 16–18.

Williams, A. (2001) A study of practising nurses' perceptions and experiences of intimacy within the nurse–patient relationship. *Journal of Advanced Nursing*, **35**(2), 188–96.

Worth, A. (2001) Assessment of the needs of older people by district nurses and social workers: a changing culture? *Journal of Interprofessional Care*, **15**(3), 257–66.

# CHAPTER 6

# The experience of a children's community nurse specialist

*Zoë Wilkes*

## Editor's introduction

There are an increasing number of specialist nurses working in the community, but because of their relatively small numbers, it is unlikely that many students will get to work with them whilst on their community placement. The term *specialist* can be used in a number of ways. Firstly, it can signify working with a specialist group of clients; secondly, it can signify the application of specialist nursing skills; and thirdly it can be used to indicate advanced skills that would not normally be associated with traditional nursing, such as physical examination and provisional diagnosis. Often the term *specialist* is not well defined in these terms, and the role may incorporate a rather blurry mixture of all three.

This chapter and the next are written by nurse specialists who have the title 'Nurse Consultant'. This is a slightly more well defined title that indicates a senior nursing role that combines practice, education and research. It is useful to read these two chapters sequentially and compare and contrast the two accounts. The first account is from Zoë, who is a Nurse Consultant in children's palliative care. Zoë never set out at the beginning of her nursing career to do this, but you can see from her account how her interest and expertise began to develop as she undertook various roles. You can also see from Zoë's account how it was important to combine increasingly specialised experience with increasing academic study. There is not such a well-defined career development structure in nursing as there is for instance in medicine, but the combination of a variety of good experience and post-registration study at degree level and beyond will enable you to explore a number of interesting possibilities.

As you read through Zoë's account, reflect on the impact that this sort of specialist role has on the care of the children and their families. As a parent I can't think of a more horrific scenario than that of one of my children becoming terminally ill. However, if this were to happen then I would want someone like Zoë looking after us as a family.

# Children's palliative care

## The background

The overall aim of my role is to act as the lead professional for children's palliative and terminal care services within Leicester, Leicestershire and Rutland by providing elements of expert practice, leadership and training, and consultancy, and advancing and developing research in this area of practice. The role is based within both the Diana Children's Community Service and the Rainbows Children's Hospice. The purpose of this is to allow the development of closer links and communication between the community and the hospice environment, along with collaborative working with the surrounding children's hospitals.

My key responsibilities are to update my own practice to ensure that it remains evidence-based and of good quality. I work closely with various members of the team to encourage development, improve practice and increase experience levels. I also take part in on-call service implemented by the Diana Service for children in the terminal stages of their disease. As a Nurse Consultant I have a leadership and training role working collaboratively with the Senior Nurse – Professional Development at Rainbows Hospice in providing study days and training packages based on children's palliative care on a national basis. We arrange conferences for multi-professional groups on the various subjects surrounding children's palliative care, working closely with professionals in this area to encourage confidence and competence.

My clinical consultancy role includes providing advice and support to all professionals caring for a child and family with palliative/terminal care needs. In addition, I provide advice and support to children and their families (including the wider family) on the subject of the child's palliative and terminal care needs. My final role is to assist in the development of research and practice by ensuring that practice is evidence-based and by keeping up to date with current research and practice (Department of Health, 2001) and by informing others of advances in research and ensuring its implementation in practice. We also aim to undertake research around the subject of children's palliative/terminal care and ensure that the findings are circulated and implemented where appropriate.

## My typical week

Although the title of my role suggests that I work with children requiring terminal care on a regular basis, this is not the case. Within both the community and the hospice, the numbers of children requiring such care are quite low most of the time (although we sometimes become quite busy following a high number of referrals at certain times of the year). The largest number of children I do come into contact with are those requiring ongoing palliative care and symptom management, who often require input at numerous times throughout the long duration of their illness. At such times I am available to offer advice and support to both professionals and the child and family, along with teaching and education around various health issues and elements.

I spend quite a lot of time developing or adapting local guidelines and policies for use within both the Hospice and the Community. I ensure they are evidence-based and in line with other community trusts and children's hospices. These are then passed through Clinical Governance Committees prior to their implementation into practice.

As a large part of my role is based on research, I commit some of my time to collecting data for a current project I am undertaking and analyse the findings to ensure their relevance to practice. I am currently writing a research strategy for Rainbows Children's Hospice in order that other members of staff may undertake their own research projects with my assistance and guidance to promote the Children's Hospice movement and develop this area of research further.

I work closely with the Professional Development nurse at the Hospice in order to establish study days and courses around the various topics within children's palliative care. I also arrange various conferences for individual professional groups to broaden their knowledge around this subject and to inform them of the various valuable resources they can currently access in order to improve care and increase parental and child choices.

I am a Basic Life Support Trainer along with one of my colleagues within the Diana Service. We teach professionals within specialist community child health services, as well as those at Rainbows, on a monthly basis. This often takes a large portion of time, as national standards and teaching guidelines must be followed in order that those attending can be deemed safely competent to undertake this form of resuscitation.

As well as arranging them, I am asked to speak at various conferences regarding many aspects of children's palliative care. Therefore some of my time is spent developing presentations and workshops in order to promote such services and increase awareness of children's palliative care.

## How did I get here?

My interest in children's palliative and terminal care began following a period of working on a paediatric intensive care unit in London nine years ago. I quickly began to establish that such care was very scarce, and that both prior to and following the death of a child there was little support for the child, family and staff involved in the care. I then moved to a brand new children's hospice situated in the heart of Kent. I joined before the hospice was open to children and families and had much input into service provision and available resources for the local families that were to use the hospice. My role of senior staff nurse was to last for three and a half years, during which I felt it important to develop my specialist knowledge, which I did by undertaking a degree in children's pain. This enabled me to gain much experience and knowledge around the symptom management of children admitted to the hospice, both for respite and terminal care. I developed a passion for this area of nursing and felt I had much to offer these children and their families, not only through my knowledge and skills, but through my newfound ability to form lasting professional relationships with them, providing continuing advice and support and learning from them of their stoic and inspiring coping mechanisms at such a sad, stressful time of their lives.

I then moved to Leicestershire where I commenced work at Rainbows Children's Hospice as the Acting Deputy Head of Care. Once again, my motivation for this work encouraged me to apply for a role within the community, caring for the same client group within their homes. This increased my job satisfaction further as I was able to recognise the importance of child and parent choice and witness the value of caring for the dying child in his or her home.

When my current post was advertised, linking both the hospice and the community, I knew it was the job for me. I was lucky enough to commence the post in January 2004 and have now completed my MSc Health Sciences along with the Extended Nurse Prescribing Course. As well as my academic qualifications, other practical and professional experiences are vitally important in developing the appropriate qualities required to undertake this particular role and consist of knowing my own limitations and when to ask for help and advice as well as recognising the need for boundaries. It is a role that enables me to become very dedicated to the children and families we are caring for, but it is important to recognise the importance of self-preservation and reflection.

Other qualities, in the form of an outgoing personality where the forming of new professional relationships becomes second nature, are vital. The families and children will look upon us as advisors and advocates. It is therefore important that we are able to dip in and out of this part of the role where necessary and where appropriate.

## Pleasures, challenges and future directions

The nurse consultant role brings with it many challenges due to the strategic levels of working required along with the implementation of various elements of practice in areas opposed to certain changes. Add to that the emotional and sensitive issues surrounding children's palliative care and the lack of research and information readily available, and the challenges become more complex. However, as the professional currently undertaking this role, these elements of challenge and complexity bring much job satisfaction and increase my motivation and enthusiasm as I work to ensure the successful completion of policy development and creation, research implementation and the continuing development of palliative and terminal care practice. Following a recent conference aimed at a certain group of professionals working with children and families in the terminal stage of illness, the increase in the knowledge and skills of the delegates was very positive (evident in both the conference evaluation and through follow-up four weeks later when application to practice was discussed). Training and education are a very important element of this role and one that I value very much. Through such responses, where confidence and competence are evidently improved (and as a result so is practice), I am inspired to continue such practice and work closely with multi-professional groups to implement and promote the same outcomes.

Another valuable element of this role is that of hands-on practice. In order to ensure that the content of teaching sessions and the evidence-based research are all up-to-date and relevant to children's palliative care, this element of the role is vital. As a lead for children's palliative and terminal care and therefore a role model for such professionals working in this area, the role is required to pioneer new developments and ensure the safe implementation of current ones. I very much enjoy this area of my work as it provides me with information regarding areas of concern, issues to be considered and evaluated and areas where good practice is being undertaken.

Some of the difficulties encountered consist of lack of time, lack of resources or funding and, as previously stated, the lack of information and research surrounding children's palliative and terminal care. These have been overcome in some instances; however, I am aware that many services and Trusts have similar issues. The lack of time element was due to the commitment to my continuing professional development, where I undertook an MSc and the extended nurse-prescribing course, which prevent me from being in practice for two days each week. This is quite frustrating when issues arise within practice and my accessibility and availability are compromised due to other commitments.

Lack of resources and funding are common problems within all areas of practice and have an effect on the number of courses attended, held and organised. However, through networking with many various professionals, I am in contact with charities and organisations that are more than willing to sponsor an event or conference or provide funding for equipment that allows us to provide terminal care for a child and their family at home. Such organisations continue to be invaluable to the development and implementation of quality palliative and terminal care. The lack of information and research within this area of practice is a problem that we as professionals can rectify. Through implementation of our own research and networking on a national and international basis, good practice can be shared, allowing for evidence-based information and knowledge to be circulated and so improving and increasing knowledge and skills within this area.

The development of this role is very dependant on the future funding of children's palliative care services. Within my own particular role, development is now based upon the completion of the courses previously stated and the implementation of these into practice. Research plays a huge part in the future of the role, as issues arise and lack of information becomes more evident. As the lead for this area of practice, it becomes my role to ensure and encourage the implementation of research and ensure such findings are accessible, not only by other professionals but also by the children and families using such services. Developments within the role may also consist of the expansion of the children's palliative and terminal care services currently provided, maybe even with another nurse consultant on board in order that specialised areas of interest, such as research or training, can be wholly adopted by one professional in order that more time can be committed to this element of practice while just as vital areas are also being considered and developed.

## Patient care

Patients cared for within the palliative care services are those children and young people living with a life-limiting or life-threatening illness and are unlikely to live into adulthood and their families. Such children consist of those with oncological conditions, neurological conditions, degenerative illnesses, cardiac conditions and those without a diagnosis but who exhibit symptoms which are deemed to be life threatening. We come into contact with such children and young people at various times throughout their illness. During the chronic palliative phase the children may be seen for issues such as symptom management, seizure control, occupational therapy and physiotherapy issues, and social and emotional issues, as well as regular visits for updates and future planning with the families. These children and their families will not be discharged from the service following such care, but instead will become inactive cases, as our input is not required during the child's 'well' phases other than to advise on schooling issues or to ensure the child's and family's emotional and social well-being are considered at all times.

As the children/young people then enter the terminal phase of their illness and nursing care becomes paramount, the teams will then become involved in ensuring that the provision of care is patient and family focused and that choices regarding the child's place of death are adhered to.

Post-bereavement support is also implemented in the form of contact from the key-worker to establish further resources and services required by the family and referral to various services in order to provide counselling or advice and support to the family.

The needs of the child/young person and the family are assessed on a continuing basis. As previously stated, during the palliative phase of the child's illness the assessment process is a continuous one (ACT, 2004) where all aspects of the child/young person's illness and life are taken into account. The impact that these may have on the family are also considered and appropriate action is implemented to ensure quality of life for not only the child but also those that care for them.

Changes to the child's condition or family circumstances require further assessment to take place, as care currently provided may now not be appropriate or beneficial to the child or family. Any professional involved in the child's care may undertake the assessments as long as they are deemed competent to do so and are fully aware of the child and family's circumstances. It is then vital that the outcome of the assessment is then communicated effectively to all other professionals involved in the child's care, in order that changes and developments may be implemented promptly to ensure that the quality of life of both the child and family remains optimal.

Assessments during the terminal phase of the child's illness are undertaken on a daily basis, or more frequently if the child's condition dictates. This is undertaken by the nurses who have frequent contact with the child and family in collaboration with the child's GP or named consultant. Changes in symptoms and medication, and any additional needs, are assessed and the necessary action is promptly taken; for example: ordering necessary equipment, alterations in drug dosages, additional medication required, changes in family circumstances, and changes of family and child's wishes. All such alterations are then communicated to all other professionals involved in the child's care and most importantly to the child and family.

# Case history

The case history (see box) is an actual account of a child and family requiring terminal care at home. In order to protect the confidentiality and anonymity of both the staff involved and the child and family, all names have been changed.

---

## Case history

Lilly is a 10-year-old girl. She lives at home with her parents, her 12-year-old brother and 15-year-old sister. When Lilly was 2 years old she was diagnosed with a malignant tumour behind her left eye. Lilly commenced treatment straight away, although due to the tumour she began to lose her sight. As her treatment began to take effect, Lilly's sight returned and the tumour reduced significantly in size. However, as Lilly progressed through her life the tumour returned on numerous occasions, requiring much intensive treatment and raising life-changing issues for both herself and her family. When the tumour reappeared as Lilly reached 10 years of age and treatment was deemed futile, her parents made a very brave decision, in collaboration with Lilly's oncology consultant, to discontinue her intensive treatment, which was making her very ill and affecting her immediate quality of life. It was not having an effect on the tumour. Lilly was discharged home under the care of the children's community nursing team while still under the care of her oncology consultant.

Prior to Lilly's discharge the community team was made aware of her diagnosis and potential prognosis and of the parents' wishes for her to pass away in the comfort of her own home. During this time, an assessment of Lilly's home was undertaken to ensure that equipment needs were considered along with issues relating to moving and handling, sleeping requirements and aids in order to maintain Lilly's dignity and quality of life. Lilly's potential medication requirements were also considered at this stage in order that pain relief and other symptoms were considered to ensure their prompt treatment as they occurred. An emergency box was taken into the home containing medication and equipment to ensure that Lilly's quality of life would be maintained, and communication with her oncology team allowed for potential symptoms to be discussed and acted upon.

Lilly's discharge date was discussed and communicated to the community team. A thorough handover from the oncology ward to the community was undertaken and on the day Lilly was discharged, a visit was carried out by two nurses from the community team to establish any further needs and introduce other members of the team.

Home visits were undertaken on a daily basis, and on occasions two visits were carried out where Lilly's condition dictated. The community team activated a 24-hour on-call service in order that her parents could contact them both during the day and out-of-hours to ensure once again that Lilly's quality of life could be maintained and her symptoms controlled. Such a service also supports parents during this phase of their child's illness, either through reassurance or the maintenance of their own self-preservation and quality of life.

Lilly remained at home with support from the community team in collaboration with her oncology consultant for a period of 13 weeks. During this time her condition deteriorated significantly, but through daily assessments and visits by the team, along with effective communication with the oncology consultant, her symptoms were managed and her family were thoroughly supported in her care.

Lilly passed away very peacefully in the arms of her mother. The community nurses on call were with her and ensured she was not in any pain or discomfort. Following her death, the nurses supported Lilly's family in bathing and dressing her and contacting her GP and oncology consultant and their chosen funeral directors. The nurses remained with the family until Lilly's body had been taken to the funeral home. They ensured that the family were ready for them to leave prior to their departure.

Contact is still maintained between the community team and Lilly's family in order to ensure they feel supported through their grief. Referrals to appropriate services have been made for both Lilly's parents and siblings to encourage self-preservation and acceptance of their grief patterns.

## Student nurses on placement

This is a very specialist placement for student nurses and one that has the potential to cause considerable stress for some students; therefore it is very important that students are chosen who have the maturity to cope with what can be a very difficult placement. For the right students this is a placement that offers tremendous experience. The learning aims are that students will learn the importance of thorough assessment throughout any phase of a child's illness through effective communication and information sharing. They will learn how to access valuable resources and equipment in order to promote a child and family's quality of life and the continuation of 'normality' at a time when this is threatened. Students will learn to do the following:

- Recognise holistic elements of palliative/terminal care.
- Recognise the importance of effective communication with multi-professionals.
- Understand the differences between palliative and terminal care.
- Have an awareness of local and national guidelines, protocols and policies in order that care implemented is evidence-based and validated.
- Have an awareness of referral procedures and criteria for all children and families referred to the service for future reference.
- Recognise the importance and the various roles of the multidisciplinary team in the palliative/terminal care of the child and family.

# Students' learning objectives

*Expectations of students on placement*

- Appearance
  - Smart/casual dress
  - Name badge must be worn at all times
- Behaviours
  - Patient confidentiality must be maintained at all times
  - Some visits may be of a very sensitive nature; therefore respect for the wishes of staff and parents must be adhered to
  - Students must maintain a professional manner at all times throughout community visits
- Interaction with patients
  - Professionalism must be maintained at all times
  - Patient confidentiality must be respected at all times
  - Be aware of sensitive situations and act accordingly
- Expected knowledge
  - Be aware of current service provision
  - Have an awareness of current issues surrounding children's palliative care
  - Have an awareness of existing policies/guidelines reflecting the provision and development of children's palliative care

## Tips for student nurses

Depending on the time of year, dress appropriately. In the summer, travelling in a hot car can be very uncomfortable if not dressed accordingly. In the winter, being outside can be very cold and damp.

Bring a map of the local area, as some visits may require you either to make your own way there or to follow the nurse to the visit (if you have your own transport).

Bring sandwiches and a number of drinks. If you are out on home visits for most of the day, you may not be near a water supply or shops. Sandwiches are also easier to eat than hot or liquid foods, as there may not be access to a microwave oven or kettle.

Wear comfortable clothing and shoes. Some locations are situated out in the country or high up within a block of flats.

Bring something to read or some work to do, as there may be occasions when visits are cancelled or the family do not wish you to enter the house.

## Editor's comments

How did Zoë's account and description of her role compare with your expectations of what that her role would entail? What areas of her role surprised you? Were you expecting a more clinical role or a less clinical one? I know approximately ten Nurse Consultants, and each of them has developed the role quite differently, depending on their initial job description, the nature of their client group and the type of nursing/medical speciality in which they work. The general remit of a Nurse Consultant is that they combine clinical work with education and research. However, this is not an easy combination, as each role is a specialist role in its own right, and expecting one individual to be a skilled clinician, teacher and researcher is asking a lot. Most of the Nurse Consultants that I know seem to combine clinical practice and teaching as the main part of their role, with the research role taking the third priority. It is early days for Nurse Consultants and it will be interesting to follow the development of the role over the next few years.

Compare Zoë's account with the account of Helen in the next chapter. Both have the title of Nurse Consultant and both work in the community, yet they have very different roles. Is this a role that you aspire to? If so, how are you going to plan your career to achieve this or a similar goal? For any such role you need to:

- Be an able clinician with excellent patient skills
- Be an expert in your area of practice
- Have a wide experience of your speciality
- Have post-registration education at degree/masters level
- Have the ability to inspire others regarding your speciality
- Have the ability to teach others
- Have the ability to participate in and possibly lead research
- Coordinate the work of others for whom you are not the line manager

This is an impressive list, and very few people will be skilled in all aspects. However, roles such as Nurse Consultants are rare and the competition is high, so aim high, but most of all try to enjoy your work. Because if you are enthusiastic and motivated about your role then this is infectious, and other people will want you to work with and for them.

# References

ACT (2004) *A Framework for the Development of Integrated Multi-agency Care Pathways for Children with Life-threatening and Life-limiting Conditions.* ACT, Bristol.

Department of Health (2001) *Research Governance Framework for Health and Social Care.* HMSO, London.

# CHAPTER 7

# The experience of working with asylum seekers

*Helen Rhodes*

## Editor's comments

Helen is the second example in this book of a nurse specialist. Her specialist area is two-fold; firstly she has advanced skills in assessment within a primary care setting and secondly she focuses on a specific client group: asylum seekers. As with Zoë, she is a Nurse Consultant and this role holds certain responsibilities. As you read through her account try to compare her role with Zoë's in the previous chapter and identify the similarities and the differences in the way that the roles have been developed to meet the needs of two very different client groups.

Helen had considerable nursing experience in a variety of different situations and cultures before taking up her current position. In some ways her career developed by chance – she could never have predicted some years ago that she wanted to become a Nurse Consultant specialising in the area of asylum seekers. This is true of many nurses in currently in senior positions. This is partly due to the fact that in the past nursing promotion was into either management or education. There were very few exciting and challenging roles that managed to combine any combination of clinical practice, education, research or management. Previously, junior nurses had very few role models, such as Helen, in terms of specialist nurses or consultant posts, and the idea of planning a career in any structured way was relatively unknown. However, in the current culture of nursing a huge variety of interesting and challenging opportunities exist, and if you are at the beginning of your career then you need to give serious thought as to what experience and post-registration education you want to gain. A significant number of these new and exciting opportunities are developing and will continue to develop in all areas of community nursing. At the heart of all such roles are the key and crucially important skills of all nurses. These are difficult to list, but include the ability to relate empathically to a broad spectrum of people, to gain their trust and assist and enable them to access and utilise health care provision. It is at times to act as an advocate, whilst at others to encourage health promotion. The clinical skills of nurses will vary depending on the area in which they are working: for some it will be wound management, for others it will be providing the activities associated with daily living, and for other group it will be counselling and listening skills. The technical expertise of different nurses will vary. However, no matter how senior we become, we will always practice with the heart and mind of a nurse. This is something we should not only cherish but be proud of. As you read through Helen's account you will see such skills demonstrated. At times this is a demonstration of advanced practice, but at the core of all her practice is the way she cares for people.

# Working with asylum seekers

## My background and the development of a unique post

I have always enjoyed my nursing career. It has been varied and opened many new and exciting opportunities for me. I also was lucky enough to work with the Aboriginal population of Australia and in the Middle East, which provided experience of working with very different cultures. This has proved invaluable to me recently. On returning to the UK, I decided that I would like to continue working in the community and was fortunate to obtain a job as a practice nurse in Leicester. I enjoyed the continuity of patient care that this role offered and I also enjoyed the diversity of the role. My interest in different cultures and their health beliefs was rekindled during the Kosovan crisis in 1999. We received mercy flights here and I was part of a team who assessed the health needs of the new arrivals; this was a challenging and fascinating experience. Asylum seekers first arrived in the city of Leicester in 2000 (Home Office, 1999). At that time very little was known about their health needs. Providing primary care has been a tremendous challenge, not at least because so little was known about this group or what their health needs were.

My original post as a clinical nurse specialist was to liaise with general practices to try to help provide services to this highly diverse group. My practice nurse background was ideal, providing a key linking role. However, it become increasingly clear that mainstream GP services were unable to deliver a service that was appropriate for this group of people. This was due to the language barriers, not understanding the way in which access and utilisation of the NHS occurred, the high use and cost of GP time, and that some of their requirements were more complex. All these things combined to make meeting their needs extremely difficult. These difficulties led to my development of a Nurse Consultant-led GP facility which provides a specialist service led by patients' needs and providing equity to access to primary care services. It provides a comprehensive and consistent approach to all aspects of health and social care to all asylum seekers within the city, and this has had a major impact on addressing health inequalities.

My key responsibilities include:

- Providing advanced clinical practice which involves assessing individuals holistically, using a range of different assessment methods and reaching valid, reliable and comprehensive client-centred conclusions which manage risk and are appropriate to needs, context and culture.
- Consulting with clients who present with undifferentiated and undiagnosed problems, making professional autonomous decisions for which I hold sole responsibility. This includes ordering investigations and independent prescribing.
- Health screening and patient education.
- Communicating with clients in ways, which empower them to make informed choices about their health and social care, and actively promote their well being.
- Undertaking audit and research to ensure that the team's service meets the needs of patients and to identify gaps in service provision within and outside the team.
- Providing clinical leadership, expert advice and support to the nursing team within the PMS and being a resource for developments of similar projects in other areas. I make a specialist nursing contribution to the strategic planning and innovative development of the service for asylum seekers and new refugees.
- In partnership with other team members, being responsible for defining, monitoring and maintaining standards of treatment and care. Benchmarking and evaluating service provision.
- Providing a lifelong learning environment to ensure the continuous professional development of other nursing team members.
- Taking a lead role in the development of the service, with effective change management, in a service where precedents do not exist.
- Working successfully in partnership to achieve a high level of inter-agency collaboration and liaison will be required to provide a holistic approach to this vulnerable group.

The Nurse Consultant role for the service reflects four key areas: expert function, leadership, research and service development. The role is 50% clinical and 50% other functions. The major clinical aspect is providing on-the-day triage for all patients, which is a key element of the service for meeting the 24 hour access targets to a health professional. The role encompasses independent assessment and diagnosis of undifferentiated diagnoses, ordering of investigations (including independent X-ray requests) and referrals to secondary care. I am an extended and supplementary prescriber. This extended role is a relatively new development in nursing and one that not every nurse would want to undertake. From my perspective, I really enjoy the extended role; it provides the opportunity to offer whole episodes of holistic care and the development of a new service is an exciting and challenging role.

This specialist service has had a very positive beginning. It is meeting the needs of an extremely vulnerable group of people, many of whom have suffered horrific forms of abuse in their home country. However, the service and my role need to continue to develop in line with patient needs using the underpinning philosophy of action research. As we seek to learn and develop from our experiences we want to make this valuable information available to others with similar needs, thus supporting and influencing local and national polices.

As all the nursing posts within my service are developmental, a large part of my role is providing mentorship and support, and through positive leadership I try to enable the rest of the nurse team to reach their potential, fulfilling their ambitions. I also provide mentoring placements for post-registration students on the Community Nursing Degree in health visiting and district nursing. The service as a whole provides a positive learning environment for numerous colleagues.

When this opportunity arose it was initially a short-term contract. It was a big risk to leave a permanent position to undertake a short-term contract with an unknown client group. However, at that time I felt I needed a change and a new challenge. Unfortunately, in the career structure of nursing it has been necessary to move away from direct patient contact if you want to progress to more senior and better paid positions. This is beginning to change, and the division between 'management', 'practice' and 'education' is no longer always so major. I feel very fortunate in that the Nurse Consultant position I have combined all three of these roles.

When I first started looking after this client group I needed to have a much greater understanding of so much, including world politics, different cultures and even geography. It was, as they say, 'a steep learning curve'. In an outreach worker role, often with no medical backup, it was clear that I would have to extend my clinical diagnostic skills. To that end I completed a postgraduate certificate in advanced diagnostic assessment and reasoning. Not only am I able to use my extended nurse skills, but this role has provided me with some exciting opportunities. Having undertaken the challenge of developing a service for a new client group, which was unique at that time, I had to gain a lot of new knowledge in many different and new areas. This has now led to some very exciting and privileged opportunities, including being able to influence health care at various levels, including working nationally and directly with the Home Office and the Department of Health. I take a major role in profiling, health needs assessment and evaluation of these clients' needs.

## Patient care

Our typical patient is a young male. They will have had to leave their home and country in a hurry, leaving everything and everyone behind. They will have had to pay a trafficker a substantial sum of money to escape and travel to a place of safety. Some will have had a protracted and hideous journey in the back of a lorry. After the initial immigration processes they will be dispersed to designated areas. On arrival they are usually disorientated, confused and understandably distressed. The physical manifestation of distress (somatisation) is frequently seen as headaches, musculo-skeletal aches and stomach upsets – these are almost universal in this client group (Izycki, 2001). When this is compounded by the stress and worry about their family and of their future, it is hardly surprising that asylum seekers are seen as high users of GP time. Sleep disturbance, including nightmares and terrors, are frequent: they occur in 28% of all asylum seekers (Hiley and Rhodes, 2005). With the manifest anxiety and distress of this client group the temptation is to label patients with mental health problems. Part of a specialist service is the expertise developed within the team, allowing the increased understanding of these symptoms of appropriate distress, and providing specialist assessment and ongoing support to keep patients well.

As well as the young men who are seeking asylum there has been a recent change to include an increase in the number of women and children. This new group brings new challenges to our service. The women are often escaping from equally horrific and traumatic experiences. The sexual assault rate seen at the service is 6.4% (Hiley and Rhodes, 2005). The service has to be able to respond quickly to changes in the profile of the population it serves.

The ASSIST service has improved access to health care by developing an integrated primary care service to meet the immediate health needs of asylum seekers and to support their transition into mainstream practice if they receive refugee status. On registration with the service all patients have an extensive health assessment, which includes a basic mental health assessment. This has been developed by our service as no precedents exist.

Marie's example (see box) demonstrates to me just how important multi-agency working and social care are, particularly with this client group who are

## Case history

Marie is 20 years old. She was looking forward to a bright future studying law. One day in December she was helping her village decorate the village for Christmas. Suddenly two lorries arrived with rebel forces. They rounded up the entire village and separated the young women from the rest. They then shot most of the others and herded the women into the trucks. She was taken to a camp and held hostage for seven months, and repeatedly sexually assaulted until she became too thin and ill and was tossed into a ditch outside the camp. She started to crawl to safety. A passing motorist picked her up and took her to the nearest village; someone there had a relative who worked for an airline. She was smuggled aboard the plane, which was coming to the UK.

I first met her when she was placed here. She was lonely, frightened and traumatised, but nevertheless I was astounded at her dignity and her composure in the circumstances. Working in partnership with our secondary care colleagues we started to address her most urgent physical needs. I could not believe how any human being could have been treated so appallingly and survive. I was distressed for several days, but you cannot dwell on what you are dealing with: you just have to focus on what can you do to help or you cannot cope personally. Just before I broke up for the holidays I asked her what else could I do for her. She wanted to attend church over Christmas. I made a few telephone calls and found a church that was willing to see what they could do. When I got back from my break I caught up with her to see how she had got on. She had had a marvellous time, although of course it reminded her exactly what she had lost. Months on, she is putting her life back together, doing voluntary work whilst awaiting a decision on whether she can stay.

often very isolated. Working closely with all the relevant agencies is essential to providing any sort of continuity of care, and the signposting for social and cultural support furthers the holistic approach that the service uses. The role could all be depressing, however; my job satisfaction is watching the clients being able to move on with their lives and start to live again. What is absolutely essential is having the time and patience to establish a trusting relationship. This we achieve by being friendly and open and providing an environment which is less imposing. We hope that this facilitates trust and confidence in the patients.

# Student nurse learning aims and opportunities

A student placement with the service provides an opportunity to gain some insight and knowledge into providing health care to a socially excluded client group. It provides an opportunity to reflect on cultural diversity and health beliefs. This is very much a specialist placement and would not suit all student nurses. Specifically, it offers:

- Consultation skills using interpreters, both face to face and via telephone links
- Consultation skills with patients who have no past medical history and who are often highly complex/confused
- Working in a GP setting with a flat hieratical management model
- Experience in working in a high skill mix service model
- Learning about different cultural health beliefs
- Active learning about patients with high levels of post-traumatic stress disorders/anxiety and mental health in a GP setting

Students on placement should be aware of some key points. When using an interpreter:

- If there is someone else is in the room do not hold other conversations at the same time or make side remarks.
- Do not use family/husband/friends to interpret.
- Always use female-to-female interpreters where possible.
- Do not forget the importance of non-verbal communication.

Also:

- I always shake their hand. This is very culturally appropriate and shows the patient respect.
- Do not assume stable family units. Extended families are common.
- Always ask what they expect. Their expectations could be very different from our agenda.
- It is important to emphasise to the patient that no information is sent to the immigration authorities without their permission.
- Trust is everything. They may be too frightened to tell you everything.
- Never promise anything you do not have total control over the delivery of.
- Next of kin issues are often a tribal concept.

# Editor's comments

I hope you found Helen's account exciting and inspiring. It is difficult for her to get over the full picture of her role – the service she provides and the way in which she provides it – in such a short account. But I'm sure you will agree that she manages to convey quite a full picture of an interesting and innovative role whilst maintaining a human quality to her account. Although it will probably be some years before you have the experience to work in such a specialised area, be sure to take every opportunity you can to go on a placement or visit people who work in these unusual areas.

As you reflect upon Helen's account think about what you can learn from her experiences and her work. At the first level there is something about being prepared to push forward the accepted role of the nurse, not for the sake of it, but to meet the needs of our patients and to move forward in a rapidly changing world. At another level there is something about being prepared to take a step of 'faith'. Going for a job that is only guaranteed for two years, not knowing everything there is to know about the job before we take it on, and being prepared to learn and learn quickly. Being prepared to direct our own learning and whilst valuing a structured course, and being prepared to become an independent and self-directed learner. At another level there is something about leadership: having a belief or vision of the way in which you see a service developing and then having the energy and passion to drive that forward. All of these are wonderful qualities that will serve you well as you progress in your nursing career. Whether you aim to be a Nurse Consultant or whether you prefer to work at a staff nurse level, vision, energy and commitment will make you valued and respected by your patients, colleagues and managers alike. So aim high, have faith and belief in yourself, be prepared to work and learn, and you will probably get there.

# References

Hiley, A. and Rhodes, H. (2005) *The ASSIST Service Annual Report.* Eastern Leicester PCT.

Home Office (1999) *The Immigration Act.* HMSO, London.

Izycki, K. (2001) A safe haven. *Mental Health Practice*, **4**(6), 12–15.

# CHAPTER 8

# The experience of working as a Health Visitor

*Karen Ford*

## Editor's introduction

Most student nurses will have a placement with a Health Visitor as part of their community placement. As a general rule about 60–75% of the Health Visitor's role is common to all and involves the standard support and developmental checks associated with the under 5s and their families. The other part of the Health Visitor's role can vary tremendously between different Health Visitors. Some may specialise in children with diabetes, some with children with special needs, some will work with older people, and others will focus 100% on the under 5s. The Health Visitor's speciality focuses predominantly on family health care in early childhood. This involves the early stages soon after a baby is born, supporting the mother by being there as a 'wise person', giving advice on sleeping – both of the baby and the parents – breastfeeding, immunisation, toileting, developmental checks, diet, play, socialisation and all the aspects of normal development. The Health Visitor is also the first contact for parents who feel that their child may not be developing in the 'normal' way. The Health Visitor will support the family as the child becomes the subject of secondary care and all the traumas that involves.

It is quite difficult to experience the breadth of the role of the Health Visitor when you may only spend a few days or a couple of weeks on placement with them. If your previous placement was on a fast-moving medical ward the contrast can seem somewhat slow and the role of the Health Visitor can seem a little vague. The skills of the Health Visitor centre on the ability to build a long-term relationship with a young family and on advocacy. As you read through Karen's account you will appreciate the breadth of her role and the subtlety of the skills that she has to enable her practice. Placements with Health Visitors are not what you might call 'exciting' in the way that working on an acute medical ward might be. Health Visitors work predominantly with healthy families, seeking to promote health and prevent illness in the future. So do not judge your placement by the 'acute' nature of the work or you will be disappointed. To maximise your placement you need to be a mature learner. Discuss with the Health Visitor the nature of the health needs within that community, the social problems of the area, families that have particular problems and the ways of engaging with people who may find the health service complex and bureaucratic.

# Working as a Health Visitor

## The aim of my role

The main aims of my post are to search for health needs in every contact with clients and to seek opportunities for health promotion. I have a duty to ensure the child's needs are paramount (Children Act 1989), regardless of the complex situations I may encounter within the family. The main responsibilities of my post are:

- To promote health by working with individuals, groups and communities
- To safeguard children in the community
- To undertake holistic assessments of the child's and family's health needs
- To practice evidenced-based care and advice
- To undertake a health needs assessment of the local community, thereby enabling the best use of resources
- Practising in a non-discriminatory way
- To target those with the greatest need to reduce health inequalities
- To screen children for developmental problems
- To support families who have children with complex needs
- Promoting and supporting breast feeding
- To find opportunities to set up groups to promote health and to educate and empower people with health problems and new parents caring for their child
- Advising parents on healthy eating from birth to five years

■ To work as part of a team – both the health visiting team and the primary health care team

■ Liaising with other agencies and building partnerships with a variety of agencies (both statutory and voluntary) with the aim of influencing and promoting the health of the community

■ To participate in immunisation programmes with children and adults

■ To undertake older persons assessments in the home and make appropriate referrals

■ To run open access and appointment style clinics to support and advise parents on aspects of caring for young children

■ To visit families at home

■ To use my qualifications as an extended nurse prescriber to benefit patients and provide a seamless service of care

■ Building a professional relationship with parents to gain their confidence, thus enabling disclosure of problems

■ Detecting and supporting women with postnatal depression

■ To keep up to date with current developments in health

■ Supporting student nurses and health visitor students on placement in the community

## How I became a Health Visitor

I worked for twenty years in adult nursing in secondary care before becoming a health visitor. This experience has proved invaluable as a foundation for a career in health visiting. The role requires a breadth of knowledge that encompasses many adult health problems as well as children's health problems. The BSc (Hons) in Community Nursing (public health nursing, health visiting) is a specialist practitioner course and requires a nurse to be qualified for at least two years before undertaking it. The nurse needs to have either a diploma or degree to access the course. I did not need to be a midwife or children's nurse before I undertook the course, as the relevant knowledge to work with children in the community is acquired throughout the course. It is a 50% theoretical and 50% practice-based course, where the student health visitor works closely with a practice mentor and also runs a small caseload. I worked after qualifying as a Health Visitor in an inner city practice and then in two county practices. The county practice where I now work has many challenges, including pockets of deprivation, rural isolation issues and child protection and drug abuse problems that are often associated with city-based practices. Another large proportion of my work involves working with women suffering from postnatal depression; this is due in part to the decline of the extended family and people relocating away from family, resulting in potential social isolation without the traditional support. The reality of health visiting in the county was quite a surprise to me after moving out of the city post.

## My role

As a health visitor I work Monday to Friday, usually 8:30 a.m. to 5:00 p.m., but this can be flexible. For example, if I have a client who works I might visit at 8:00 a.m. or 5:30 p.m. so that my service adapts to their needs, rather than the other way round. I do work on some evenings: for example, I run ante-natal classes for prospective parents between 7:00 and 9:00 p.m. on two evenings per month. By using this flexible approach to working it enables the group to have many fathers attend who would normally be working if the class was held during the day; working women can also attend. The classes are part of collaborative working with the community midwife. This takes place in the health centre. The midwife runs two of the sessions and I run two as part of a rolling programme. My two sessions address breast feeding and many aspects of caring for their new baby, such as cot death prevention, nappy hygiene, adjusting to the lifestyle change and immunisations. Every two months I organise a course for new parents to teach them basic life support techniques. Again, this runs during an evening to ensure both parents can attend. These sessions are led by a firefighter who is qualified to teach infant and child basic life support. My role is one of facilitator for the group, but I also speak about managing choking in a young child. My organisational role entails sending out the appointments and I had to initially approach a local charity to gain funding to pay the firefighter; I promoted the group through the local newspaper.

There are some aspects of my work that are core work, for example certain clinics for developmental assessments, weekly open access clinics or immunisation clinics. The rest of the work is determined by the clients' needs, such as a new baby being born or a client ringing me with a problem. I also run health promotion groups and these will be on certain days within the week.

## My typical week

During a typical week I will visit families for the first time where a new baby has been born, taking over from the midwife at 11–14 days after the birth. The parents are telephoned to make a suitable appointment. The visit lasts around one hour, but anything is possible at a visit. As part of the role a health visitor has to be prepared for anything and to put aside their agenda when faced with a crisis such as a tearful mother, or a developmental concern that needs urgently referring to the GP. As a consequence, flexibility is important to respond appropriately to the client's needs. It is impossible to carry on with the Health Visitor agenda – such as trying to persuade a client to give up smoking – if they have just found out that their partner has left them and they have three children under five years and feel that they need a cigarette to help them cope. The focus of the visit would change to support, guiding them through practical issues, such as where to seek legal advice and what benefits they could access to ensure they had money for food. Also, I would listen to the woman and help her express her feelings. It may be that in time, and by providing this supportive relationship, a point will come when the woman feels she can address smoking cessation. A lack of sensitivity to her position could alienate her to a point where the woman could refuse to grant me access to her home.

During a straightforward new birth or primary visit I would listen to the parents' account of the birth, offering clarification of anything that arose from that experience. It also gives me an indication of the level of emotional trauma the mother may have experienced and alerts me to a potential postnatal depression risk factor. It will give me a basis for my visiting pattern and the degree of support that is required. I will conduct a developmental examination of the baby, weighing the child and measuring its head circumference. This information is entered in the parent-held record. I would assess the progress of the feeding method and support the parents with any problems and offer advice. Any concerns I have will be discussed sensitively with the parents, and the GP's support will be enlisted. The visit often involves dispelling anxiety over sleeping or feeding worries. I need to exercise patience by listening to the parents and respecting how they feel, offering practical solutions backed by research-based evidence. This has to be done in a way that promotes their confidence and empowers them as new parents.

The mother's health is assessed as well as that of the immediate family at this first visit. Because I will be having contact with this family over the next five years I do not have to cram everything into one visit. I can afford to tailor the information to what they can manage, especially if they have had very little sleep, knowing I will have other opportunities to promote health and address other issues that I may have discovered at another occasion. I have to ensure that I record my assessment accurately to facilitate this and keep contemporaneous records. The visit is also recorded in the parent-held record, so the parents can refer to it when any advice is offered at a later time. The information should be clear and written in a way that the individual family can understand, e.g. avoiding medical jargon. There is some paperwork to complete, such as the registration form for the GP and discussing and obtaining consent for immunisations when the baby is two months old.

During the visit I also assess the environment, such as safety in the home – is there a dog who is allowed to roam freely near the baby? Is the house in a sanitary condition? These factors can affect the health of the child and the family and need assessing. I would ascertain whether the parents have financial problems or have local support from family and friends. This is part of my preventative role – to pre-empt problems and instigate advice, offer benefit information, and provide vigilance for the future – and it will inform my visiting frequency if there are unresolved issues with which the family needs support. Some of these areas can be very sensitive and I cannot ask them in a prescriptive 'tick list' sort of way. I need to be diplomatic and find some of the information through normal, but guided, conversation. It could be suggested that a health visitor is a 'busy body', but I have a duty to protect the well-being and safety of the child and to act on their behalf to optimise their growth and development (Children Act 2004). This relaxed but directed approach takes experience to achieve. Some of the techniques are taught on the health visiting course, but putting the skills into practice is where the real learning begins. I have to reflect after each visit with a family to consider how well the visit went. It may be that I felt the conversation ran into a problem and I need to consider different ways to explain or ask a question in a similar situation. By working in the countryside I have the good fortune to drive between visits where I can debrief myself before the next visit and reflect on what has just occurred.

During my typical week I could undertake many primary or follow-up visits to support a family with a new baby. I will have visits pre-booked to support parents with a variety of issues, such as: feeding; advice on weaning their baby; toddler problems of behaviour or faddy eating; developmental problems that the parent may have detected; developmental assessments; and any subsequent referrals to other health professionals such as speech and language, audiology or the community paediatrician. I will visit clients for smoking cessation, offering a package of support including counselling support and nicotine replacement prescriptions. There will be visits to families living in poverty, lone parents and teenage parents, mainly offering support and advice and always working with the parents to promote health and improve the health and well-being of their children.

Child protection underpins much of my work. It is something I have to be constantly vigilant about, whatever social class the client is from. It is a difficult part of the role, where I have to be open with the parent and tell them of my concerns and the subsequent referral that has to be made to social services. I find my training and experience as a Health Visitor helps tremendously with this aspect of my work, giving me the confidence to tackle these difficult problems, utilising my knowledge of child protection procedures and the referral criteria. I also have a supportive team who provide clinical supervision to help me reflect on these situations, and access to a child protection lead nurse who can offer advice when I feel unsure of what action to take or how to word my report. This part of the role involves a lot of liaison with a variety of agencies and very detailed and factual record-keeping. Regular updates on a variety of child protection topics or a basic refresher course are essential for me to continue to do my job effectively, and my Trust provides this training. I also have to attend case conferences and core group meetings as part of the child protection policy if a child is put onto the child protection register. The parents also attend these meetings, which is one of the reasons I have to be open with them from the outset, but it is also laid down in the Children Act 1989 that they are consulted and involved. Child protection cases can be very emotive and I have to learn to manage this part of my work. They can also be extremely rewarding when things improve for the child and the family returns to functioning successfully through the hard work of the multi-agency team. Or the reward may be when a child is placed in a safe home away from the perpetrator of the abuse, knowing that the child is now safe.

Some of the home visits involve supporting adults with their problems, such as relationship difficulties, chronic illness, domestic violence or postnatal depression. This requires knowledge of the referral pathways that are appropriate for this particular client and situation as well as listening and support skills from the Health Visitor. My previous experience in secondary care as a general nurse has given me the knowledge and skills to deal with many aspects of my work. I feel that a Health Visitor needs to have a breadth of life experiences and a sound general nursing background to undertake this role. Some may argue that a Health Visitor should also be a parent to enable them to empathise effectively. This has been invaluable to me in being able to appreciate what it feels like to breast feed; being so tired and caring for the new baby; the challenge of toddlers or having postnatal depression; and many other felt experiences. However, when I was an intensive care sister I felt that I offered the best care possible to a patient undergoing a liver transplant although I had not experienced this first hand.

During the week I will be involved in immunising babies, toddlers and teenagers as part of the universal immunisation programme. These contacts also offer many opportunities for health promotion and I try to utilise these wherever possible. A teenager at an immunisation clinic may ask for advice about contraception; the mother of a four-year-old attending for pre-school boosters may be worried about their child's bed wetting; or I might be dealing with a four-month-old baby, attending for its third set of primary immunisations, who has eczema and requires a prescription and management advice for this condition. Sometimes a future home visit or clinic appointment is required to undertake the appropriate time to deal adequately with the problem.

All of my contacts with children involve the utilisation of the common assessment framework. This ensures that the child's developmental needs, the environmental factors and the family functioning aspects are considered. This framework enables many elements that impact on a child's health to be taken account of, and is used by a variety of agencies, such as social services, education and the police, to ensure that we work in the same way, considering the same elements that can affect a child.

Another aspect of my work which I really enjoy is the health promotion group work. This area of the role depends on the identified needs of the local community and the commitment and enthusiasm of the health visitor to set up and run the groups. I have to find a venue to hold the group, such as church hall or a nursery. I run groups for new parents to provide an opportunity to give them new research-based information and a forum for them to ask questions and make new friends. The sessions run over a six-week programme of topics and the new group can then keep in touch afterwards. This can greatly reduce their risk of postnatal depression by creating new support networks amongst their peer group and dispelling worries early on. Another group involves supporting women with postnatal depression – this is a joint venture with a local voluntary organisation, Homestart, the community mental health team and complementary therapists.

The weekly clinic offers an access point for parents to 'drop in' with their babies and children for advice on feeding issues or minor ailments. It is a busy place that also acts as a social venue for parents and again helps reduce isolation that can come with being a new parent and giving up work, or having newly moved to the area. I have to ensure I concentrate at these clinics, as I may see up to 25 people in less than two hours. I need to write on a duplicate record form, putting one in the parent-held record for the parents to utilise and remind them of the advice given and to act as my contemporaneous record. This ensures that I do not forget the detail of the contact. I see a colleague's client and this facilitates communication between us after the clinic. The clinic setting is often the time when I write the most prescriptions for minor ailments or eczema, and again this requires concentration for safe practice.

During the week there may be a professional meeting; this involves the health visiting team, nursery nurses and children's nurses. It is an opportunity for the whole team, in my case 18 of us, to meet and cover common problems and to get updates on new information or courses. Community nurses who have been on courses give a presentation on the topic, and it can be a place for one of us to give a small presentation on a researched topic that will affect us all, enabling us to update our knowledge base.

Other challenges associated with being a health visitor involve finding houses in small villages where the house only has a name and no number. It is perk of the role to work in the countryside, where I can drive through beautiful scenery and reflect on my previous visit and what action I am going to take about a problem or, if I felt that the visit did not go well, why this might be. I might be visiting a travelling family in their caravan, and the next visit could be to a family living in a mansion – this happened recently when I had a Child Branch Student with me on placement, and I used this to illustrate the diversity of the clients that a Health Visitor has to work with. It can be very challenging dealing with many phone calls when I am in the office and need to write reports following a visit. Many clients ring with minor problems, but I have to remind myself that they are big problems to them and require tact and understanding.

When a child being assessed does not achieve its developmental milestones, this is a demanding time. It requires a variety of referrals to many other health professionals as part of the assessment process. This means lots of letter writing and liaising with a variety of disciplines within the health arena, or with professionals from the education services. The parents will be very anxious and require a lot of support before a diagnosis can be made. It is an area of the job which is also very rewarding when the multidisciplinary team are working together and the child makes progress. It gives me a real sense of job satisfaction when children receive the appropriate care to optimise their potential, knowing that I have been the initial instigator in starting the process to provide that help. The work does not stop there, although other specialist services are set in motion. In the early days of the family not having a diagnosis or knowing what the long-term outcome will be for their child, my role is one of support. I provide listening visits and ensure that the family have access to information, sometimes working in an advocacy role or chasing up appointments and reducing communication problems. I strive to provide a seamless service for the family while they are coming to terms with the developmental problems that their child is exhibiting.

## My role with students

I sometimes have student health visitors with me on placement. They work with their primary mentor and I will be one of the associate mentors, providing a different perspective on the skills that a Health Visitor uses. It is important for them to experience a variety of Health Visitors at work to enable them to reflect on what they see and decide on how they will utilise the various skills and approaches when they become qualified Health Visitors.

I have student nurses more regularly on placement with me. These students are undertaking the Common Foundation Programme and experiencing their first taste of community nursing. They spend a week with a Health Visitor and a school nurse. It is challenging to provide an experience in such a short period that gives them the full range of variety of health visiting. I suggest that the aim for this short placement is to focus on families living in their normal environment and utilise this insight when they return to secondary care to improve their discharge planning. It is also an opportunity to see essentially healthy children and gives an overview of issues that can impact on them. The health visiting principles that underpin the role (Twinn and Cowley, 1991) are very clear about the effort that is needed to make a difference to the family.

Students who are undertaking the Child Branch of either the BSc (Hons) in Nursing or the Diploma in Higher Education in Nursing also spend a longer period of time with the Health Visitor and school nurse in their community nursing module. This placement is for 300 hours and offers a greater opportunity for the student to see many aspects of the work of the health visitor. I would expect the students to appreciate the opportunities for health promotion whilst on their placement. They will also see at first hand how safeguarding children happens in practice, and this will increase their knowledge of child protection procedures and identifying risk.

Students working in the community do not need to wear a uniform. Instead I would expect them to dress smartly, remembering that they are guests in the client's home. It would be disrespectful to wear high fashion that offends or extremes of makeup, piercing or hairstyles. I would expect students to show their professionalism in their dress and demeanour when communicating with clients. It may also be practical to wear comfortable shoes if a lot of walking is involved in the placement. It can be difficult in the early weeks of the placement for students observing the specialist nurse at work and not having the more practical approach they are used to in secondary care. Students need to be aware that the Health Visitor is undertaking complex assessments of need and developmental issues, utilising a variety of approaches to facilitate this. It is often only when students and Health Visitors reflect on a visit that some of the subtler issues are revealed to the students. As their placements progress, students will be invited to participate in aspects of measuring children, sometimes to participate in health promotion group work or to design and set up a health promotion display in the clinic or surgery. Students will also have the opportunity to observe a variety of agencies and professionals at work within the multidisciplinary and multi-agency teams. Students would be encouraged to relate their past nursing experiences and theoretical knowledge to the various experiences they have in practice, and to demonstrate their understanding and interest. Lots of questions are also very welcome to show the Health Visitor that students are interested in the work, questioning what is happening and relating it to the theoretical component of the module, and also to challenge the mentor.

## Editor's comments

How would you sum up the role of the Health Visitor based upon your placement experience and your reading of Karen's account? It certainly involves the under 5s and health promotion, but it is not easy to define the exact way in which this is always achieved. I hope you are beginning to appreciate the breadth and complexity of the role. It is another specialised role for the nurse and at times within the profession's history its connection to nursing has been debated. Some people have questioned whether you need to be a nurse prior to undertaking the Health Visiting course, and whether it should instead be more like a social worker's training, with a direct entry into a three-year degree programme. Most Health Visitors, like Karen, find their previous nursing experience extremely valuable, not simply for the technical skills they might bring to the role, but for the social skills, the nurse–patient relationship skills, the experience of life, and the experience of secondary care. From the client's perspective it is also extremely valuable in that people relate to and trust nurses in ways that they do not with social workers and other non-health professionals. So the background of nurse training provides a very strong base for the development of the somewhat difficult to define health visiting skills.

# Reference

Twinn, S. and Cowley, S. (1991) *Principles of Health Visiting: a Re-Examination*. Health Visitors Association, London.

# CHAPTER 9

# The experience of a primary care mental health worker

*Tony Scarborough*

## Editor's introduction

One of the biggest differences that I have noted between working in the community and working in a hospital concerns the way in which patients view nurses. If a person is admitted to hospital it is usually for one specific medical condition: a heart attack, a severe infection etc. Patients view their nurses as particularly knowledgeable in that area of illness and as a general rule both the nurse and the patient focus on the medical problem that has led to the hospital admission. In the community, however, there seems to be a significant difference in how patients perceive nurses and how nurses perceive patients – this is summed up by the word *holistic*. If you go into a patient's home with the prime intention of redressing a leg ulcer, then you will rarely simply enter the house, explain to the patient what you are going to do, carry out the dressing and leave. This might be the seemingly efficient way that a dressing in a hospital is carried out, but in the community it is usually different. You go in and explain about the dressing procedure. The patient then starts talking about her family and how isolated she feels. You ask her about her mobility and when she last went out and who does her shopping, and you ask what her diet is like and advise her on certain foods and moderate exercise. She realises that her mood is rather low and you ask about her sleep pattern and energy levels. You note that she appears a little unkempt. She confides in you that she has felt very isolated since her husband died two years ago and recently she has begun to feel increasingly low. Although you are not a psychiatric nurse, you recognise the early signs of possible depression.

Patients normally meet community nurses on a one-to-one basis, often in the privacy of their own home or a private room in a health centre. This induces an atmosphere in which the patient feels at the centre of the consultation, unlike the hospital atmosphere, where they see themselves as one of many in the ward, with nurses rushing around doing essential jobs – too busy to spend 'quality time' with them. Thus in the community patients feel freer to air their concerns and worries, not only about their specific medical problem (e.g. the leg ulcer), but also about their general health and life issues as well.

Experienced community nurses will empathise with this observation, and it is often one of the reasons why community nurses find their work so rewarding, in that they can relate to and provide holistic health care to their patients. They will also have developed sophisticated social skills that enable them to relate positively to their patients and assess and treat them as holistically as possible, yet at the same time employ strategies that extract themselves politely from conversations about the patient's son who lives in Australia, 'and by the way I have a photo album of the grandchildren, let me show it to you!' without appearing rude or dismissive.

What this means in terms of health care is that the community nurse will often pick up early symptoms of other health problems that can be treated before they become serious. This is particularly true in terms of mental health. Thus many patients will present to their GP or community nurse either with an overt mental health problem or with a physical problem which has psychological overtones. Whilst some of these problems can be dealt with by the nurse or GP, few GPs or community nurses have either the training or time to deal with these issues. The majority of these people do not need the services of the full psychiatric services and psychiatrists, and many would not like the stigma that they feel such a referral might bring. Hence the development of primary care mental health services. This provides the services of an experienced mental health care worker within a GP practice, to which patients who would benefit from short-term consultations would benefit. The therapist can see patients within the surgery, thus removing the stigma of 'psychiatric out-patients' and hopefully increasing attendance and compliance. Also, if the therapist is physically present within the surgery once a week then the other staff within the practice can use them as a resource. This is the role that Tony Scarborough has, that of a senior practice therapist. He spends half a day in different GP surgeries or health centres seeing patients or advising staff. As you read through Tony's account, think about the benefits of having someone like Tony easily accessible to community nurses.

# The experience of a primary care mental health worker

## The background

It has been estimated that over 90% of all mental health care takes place within primary care and that over a third of all general practice consultations have a significant mental health component (Department of Health, 1999). The aim of my current post is to provide access to 'talking treatments' for people with common mental health problems, such as depression and anxiety, in a primary care setting. In addition, I act as a resource for GPs and other primary care staff on issues to do with mental health and mental health promotion.

The key responsibilities of this post are:

- Assessment of mental health problems
- To provide ongoing therapeutic interventions for patients in primary care using evidenced-based psychological treatments such as cognitive behaviour therapy (CBT)
- To provide advice to GPs when referral to another mental health service is appropriate
- To signpost patients to other sources of support within the health, social care, education or voluntary sectors
- Supervision and line management of staff within the service

## My typical week

As a Senior Practice Therapist, 50–60% of my time is involved with direct patient contact. My week can be seen as ten half-days or ten sessions. Each week I spend at least five sessions in different GP surgeries, seeing approximately five patients per session. These are patients who have been referred by a GP in that practice. I see patients with a wide range of presenting problems, and the purpose of the first meeting is usually to assess the nature of the problem and whether ongoing appointments with myself are indicated or whether some other intervention may be helpful.

Each clinic comprises five appointments of 30 minutes duration. I allow myself time between appointments to write notes and prepare for the next patient. Whilst at the surgery I also take the opportunity to meet informally with

GPs, practice nurses and any other clinical or administrative staff who are at the surgery. This is an opportunity to liaise with GPs regarding any patients that they may wish to discuss and also to share information about resources, study events etc. In general, my aim is to raise awareness regarding mental health and related issues.

The rest of the week – the other five sessions – is taken up with a number of other activities. This includes receiving clinical and managerial supervision from my line manager and providing the same for the two practice therapists I line manage. Regular supervision is important, as there is a high volume of clinical work undertaken each week. Supervision can help a practitioner to manage the emotional impact of meeting with patients who may be in a state of distress or who may be talking about traumatic and abusive past experiences. Supervision can also provide ideas for a way forward with work that may appear to be 'stuck'.

In addition I attend team meetings. There is a weekly meeting for all my colleagues working within the PCT. The meeting serves many functions. There is an opportunity for peer supervision where clinical material is discussed and many ideas can be generated about constructive interventions. Journal articles are also discussed. This provides a useful forum for sharing opinions and form- ing ideas based on current research or policy issues. Sometimes visiting speak- ers from other projects or agencies may attend the meeting to keep us updated on developments. Recent visitors have come from a new Connexions outreach project which aims to support young people (up to 24 years) who are not cur- rently in employment, education or training. We also had a presentation from a Children's Fund project aiming to support mothers and children who have been affected by domestic violence.

There is a regular meeting for myself and senior colleagues with the head of service. This is largely a business meeting with a focus on service development and clinical governance issues.

The remainder of my week is taken up with a variety of activities. I often meet staff from other services to tell them about my service or to find out about theirs. I also attend the local multi-agency mental health promotion group each month and sit on the steering group of a Next Step project which supports people with common mental health problems back into work, training etc. Some time is also taken up reading and responding to a steady flow of emails and other written material.

## How I came into this job

To become a Practice Therapist it is necessary to have a 'core' mental health qualification – i.e. mental health nursing, occupational therapy, social work or psychology. In addition, the job requires a minimum of eight years post-registration experience in a recognised mental health setting where there is an emphasis on psychological/therapeutic interventions. After qualifying as a mental health nurse, my subsequent experience was gained within specialist in-patient adult mental health settings and in a community-based child and adolescent mental health service.

It is important to have a significant level of experience in a secondary care setting in order to understand the mental health service system and to be able to assess which patients can be managed appropriately within primary care and at what point referral to other mental health services may be indicated. An example of a patient who needed a referral was a 58-year-old woman of Ugandan origin. The GP referred her to me as he felt the patient had been depressed since the death of her husband four years previously. However, on meeting the patient it gradually became apparent that she was exhibiting some very fixed, apparently delusional beliefs. For example she believed her neighbour could somehow read her thoughts and she could hear the neighbours whispering about her in the middle of the night. She also believed that her former employers were circulating malicious rumours about her around the locality and to relatives in Uganda and also listening in to her phone calls. The patient was very distressed by these beliefs and was asking for help. She agreed to a referral to a psychiatrist. Being an experienced practitioner is also important in establishing the service with GPs, who need to feel confident that patients are being managed appropriately. As there is no psychiatrist attached to the CMHPS, the medical responsibility remains with the GP.

In contrast to secondary care, where I worked as part of a multidisciplinary team with other mental health professionals, this role is much more isolated. I am generally working in GP surgeries where there are no other staff with a mental health qualification. This means I need to be confident in my assessments and interventions and be able to make decisions without immediate recourse to other colleagues.

In order to be able to work effectively in this role it is important to be able to manage the often high level of demand in terms of numbers of referrals. This involves being able to judge when to offer ongoing involvement, and for how long, and when to offer no further appointments after the initial assessment (Perris, 2003). One needs to be able to gauge quickly whether a patient's presenting problems are likely to be amenable to a talking-based approach and whether the patient is motivated enough to make use of the therapy on offer. It is also important to be aware of one's own limitations, both professionally and personally and to seek support when necessary.

It is important to be flexible in one's approach to try as much as possible to respond to the mental health needs of the patient whilst recognising the limits of what can be achieved in this setting. It is important to be able to draw upon a range of psychological concepts and treatment models and not stick rigidly to one formula or approach.

# What I like about the role

I enjoy working in a primary care setting as it can be seen as a more normalising experience for patients. I enjoy being able to introduce psychologically based interventions in primary care. These give patients a choice and where appropriate an alternative to anti-depressant medication. Having extra time for each consultation I am able to undertake a more comprehensive assessment compared with the GP, who is often limited to 5–10 minutes. I enjoy meeting a range of patients, some with longstanding, multiple issues affecting mental health (e.g. childhood abuse, domestic violence, unsatisfactory educational experience and attainments etc.). On other occasions, patients present with short-term problems linked to a specific incident or set of circumstances. Many patients can gain some degree of benefit from a few sessions – this leads to a high throughput of patients and avoids the feeling of being stuck with a long-term, unchanging caseload, which can be the case in a secondary care setting.

Another satisfying aspect of the role is being able to work in a number of different surgeries with a variety of GPs and other staff. Initially I felt like an outsider, but over a period of time good working relationships have been established with clinical and administrative staff in the various surgeries. This has now reached the stage where I feel 'at home' in the different settings without being a permanent enough fixture to be drawn into any local politics or the dynamics of different staff groups. Certainly I have been able to establish regular dialogue with GPs, something which has generally been lacking between primary care and mental health services in recent years.

# The difficulties and challenges

One of the main challenges of the job is to establish mental health as a priority issue in primary care. This is not easy due to the competing demands of the management of other illnesses and conditions within this setting. In addition, staff who have little or no formal training in mental health may not feel confident in the assessment and management of mental health problems and also may not appreciate the potential within their role in terms of mental health promotion. Staff in primary care, such as practice nurses, are in an important position in terms of mental health and part of my task is to support them in this function.

Another difficulty to be addressed is that of non-attendance of patients, both for initial assessments and follow-up appointments. One of the reasons for establishing mental health services in primary care is to make services more accessible, less stigmatising and more acceptable to patients. The target for the service is to have a non-attendance rate below 15%, and in many surgeries this is achieved. However, in some surgeries this figure is exceeded, probably due to a number of factors. One issue we have identified is the need for GPs to avoid crisis-driven referrals. Often if people are referred when in a state of immediate distress they may decide not to attend once the situation has settled. I generally advise GPs to see patients for a follow-up to see if problems persist before considering referral to the common mental health problem service. My task is to discuss cases with GPs where possible to help clarify how best to proceed.

## Future developments

The role, although relatively new, is now becoming well established in terms of clinical work. GPs generally are using the service frequently and are appreciative of the support provided. A recent patient survey also indicated a high level of patient satisfaction with the service provided. Future clinical developments could involve the establishment of more group, rather than individual, interventions. It would also be interesting to explore the possibilities of using telephone-based consultations, which is something some GPs are experimenting with. This may be useful in surgeries where there is a high level of demand for the service.

Other developments are likely to be driven by Government directives – particularly the need for Primary Care Trusts to employ Graduate Mental Health Workers and Gateway Workers (Bower, 2002). Locally the PCTs have commissioned our service to fulfil the functions of these new workers. In effect, this will mean that in addition to my substantial clinical remit, my role will expand to cover more activities regarding mental health promotion and signposting. This will involve an increasing need for inter-agency networking and liaison activities.

Another development due to legislative changes will be the expansion of the service from a 'working age adult' (16–64 years) service to a service without an upper age limit. Under new legislation, restrictive age limits are no longer acceptable and over 65s will have access to the service. The challenge for the service and referrers will be to incorporate the as yet unknown increased level of demand for the service within existing resource levels. There are also implications for staff training in assessment and interventions with more elderly patients.

# A sample of my morning's work in one clinic

To give a flavour of the work I do I will describe one clinic at an outer city practice. There are four GPs in the practice with a population of approximately 9,000 patients. The area is predominantly white working class, with a small ethnic minority population including some asylum seekers and refugees. I have one clinic session per week at the surgery.

### Patient 1

Mr A is 29 years old and unemployed. Whilst recently serving a three-month prison sentence for a domestic violence incident, Mr A was advised by a prison nurse to seek help for 'anger management'. This is my third appointment with Mr A, and we are still really in the assessment stage. Mr A reports a harsh child-hood with a father and grandfather who tended to be violent on occasions and who both had criminal records for violent offences. Mr A started using drugs (amphetamines, LSD) at age 14 and stopped attending school at that point. He has never kept a job for long and has served several short prison sentences for a variety of assault and theft offences. He currently has a partner and they have a young child. There has recently been a social services case conference due to concerns about the mother's drug use and violence between the couple. The child has been placed on the child protection register as being 'at risk of neglect'. Mr A reports no longer using illicit drugs, although he drinks alcohol regularly and is prescribed diazepam by the GP.

At present I am still assessing the potential for any change. Mr A tends to view most of his difficulties as being due to the actions of others rather than himself, although he does acknowledge that his reaction can exacerbate situa-tions. Since the birth of his child he wishes to gain more control over his temper and to obtain a permanent job. Together we are currently starting to think about some problem-solving strategies and have arranged to meet again.

### Patient 2

Mr D is 44 years old and unemployed. I had met Mr D for two appointments a few months previously – he had then failed to attend the follow-up. At that time he was reporting a moderate level of depression with a disturbed sleep pattern, lack of motivation and loss of pleasure in activities. It appeared this was connected to physical health problems: he had developed fibromyalgia and had been forced to give up his job as a plasterer. He also has relationship difficulties. His marriage of 10 years duration had ended five years previously, and there were currently difficulties in the relationship with his latest partner. At that time I introduced some CBT strategies for managing depression (Gilbert, 2002). We particularly focused on activity scheduling and re-establishing a sleep pattern.

More recently, difficulties had escalated due to the ending of his relationship – he had started drinking more in response to this and had been arrested by the police for harassing his ex-partner whilst drunk. At that point he was expressing suicidal ideas and was seen by the Crisis Team for a brief period. He has now returned to myself for ongoing assistance. He has been prescribed antidepressants and has reduced his alcohol intake. I referred him to an employment project to help develop other employment opportunities compatible with his current physical health problems. We also looked at alternative coping strategies which did not involve alcohol and arranged to meet again.

### Patient 3

Mrs J is a 26-year-old married woman with two children. Following the birth of her second child five years ago she experienced a period of postnatal depression. Her mood eventually lifted, but she was left with a generally raised level of anxiety. This had become increasingly problematic and she had developed increasing agoraphobic symptoms and panic attacks and had been prescribed beta blockers by the GP. Today is the fifth appointment.

The initial assessment identified that Mrs J had developed an exaggerated fear of dying. This was linked to the palpitations she experienced as a result of her anxiety, which she misattributed to serious heart problems. The initial intervention with Mrs J had been an educative approach outlining a CBT model of anxiety and panic, highlighting the role of cognitive distortions, catastrophic thinking, the effects of adrenaline and over-breathing. A handout was given for the patient to refer to at home.

Mrs J was well motivated to overcome her problems and having grasped the fundamental aspects of the CBT model was willing to participate in a programme of graded exposure to feared situations. We would jointly agree a series of tasks, which included going to the local shops, going to the park with her sister and children, and travelling on a bus. These were all things she had been avoiding or felt unable to do. At each session we would review tasks successfully completed and discuss any problems that had arisen. Overall Mrs J has made considerable progress and is now functioning much more effectively than previously. However, she still feels some level of anxiety and is reluctant to discontinue the beta blocker medication. Following today's appointment we agreed to meet again in two months to ensure that progress is maintained.

### Patient 4

Ms P is a 29-year-old single parent with three children. She had consulted her GP with a variety of problems following the end of a seven-year relationship characterised by high levels of domestic violence. Ms P reported feeling depressed and suffering low self-esteem. I have met Ms P on a total of ten occasions. We met six times last year, at the end of which she reported feeling a lot better – she had established a new relationship and was generally managing the children more effectively. These sessions had focussed on practical parenting issues, obtaining a job and general self-esteem raising. The approach taken was solution-focused brief therapy (George *et al.*, 1999) – this involves identifying strengths, competencies, coping abilities, exceptions to problems, best hopes for the future and so on.

However, Ms P had returned to the GP again following episodes of violence in her current relationship. She reported strong feelings of anger which had on occasion developed into physical violence against her partner. This worried her a great deal, and she had been wondering about the links between her childhood and her current difficulties in forming and maintaining healthy relationships. She described a childhood marked by neglect and emotional abuse, which had left her feeling very angry towards her mother. She experienced her mother, who had a series of partners, as very cold, emotionally distant and extremely punitive in her attempts to manage the behaviour of her seven children. Ms P now believes that her feelings of anger towards her mother tend to 'spill over' into other relationships. We are currently thinking more about these feelings and developing ways of managing them more effectively. She and her partner are currently awaiting an appointment with Relate to try to work together on building their relationship. I have also put Ms P in touch with a Women's Aid group for women who have experienced domestic violence which focuses on self-esteem and relationship issues.

### Patient 5

Mr V is a 19-year-old man. He attended the appointment following a consultation between his mother and the GP. His mother had expressed concern about her son's emotional state and the GP had suggested referral to this service. Mr V reported a traumatic experience that had occurred ten months previously. At that time he had found his girlfriend's father hanged at his girlfriend's home. The suicide was apparently completely unexpected. Immediately after this event Mr V had been troubled by sleep disturbance, flashbacks, irritability and poor concentration, and had taken two weeks off work. Over the following months he reported a general lessening of symptoms and a resumption of normal functioning. However, his relationship with his girlfriend then ended when she found a new partner. The end of this relationship had affected Mr V very considerably and he had been distressed and angry at the way it had ended. There were now signs that he was starting to move on with his life. He had been attending work regularly and had enrolled on a staff development course. He had re-established contact with some former college friends and was developing some social activities. He seemed to be gradually readjusting to the loss of what had been a very significant three-year-relationship which came on top of the trauma described earlier.

Mr V was appreciative of the time spent thinking about his situation and we jointly agreed that no further appointment necessary. We concluded that Mr V would contact his GP again in future if he thought any further help was needed.

These accounts give some indication of the types of scenarios and issues addressed during the course of a single clinic and the range of responses/interventions offered.

## Student nurse placements

As the service is relatively new we have only had a small number of students on placement to date. Mental health branch students have been placed here as their final specialist placement and have found it an extremely valuable experience. The aim of the placement is to gain an understanding of mental health care provision in a primary care setting, to identify social, environmental and family factors which may dispose towards the development of a mental health problem and to be aware of the range of brief interventions which can help in the management of those problems.

During the placement students would be expected to participate in mental health promotion activities by networking with other agencies and by advertising local resources within the surgery. By the end of the placement, having observed practice therapists at work, the student will be able to conduct an initial interview with a patient under supervision.

I would expect the students to dress in a smart but casual way. Extreme fashions can be off-putting to a number of patients and it is important to be able to build up a trusting relationship in a relatively short period of time. It is always useful if students bring a packed lunch with them and a book or journal to read when there are periods of inactivity. Generally the experience is very interesting for the students, but some may find the relatively slower pace, compared to an admission ward, a little difficult to adjust to. If you as a student feel that this might apply to you, then try to appreciate what is happening within the consultations and within the scenario of primary care.

## Editor's comments

The development of mental health workers as part of the primary care team is a relatively new development for the NHS. Previous roles have always been as a satellite service of the in-service psychiatric team. This development gives greater autonomy to the practice therapist and allows for greater inter-professional working with the primary health care team. Not all of the practice therapists have a nursing background: some are psychology graduates who have undergone a postgraduate mental health workers course. The main aim of such a role is to provide early and appropriate intervention to people who are experiencing some form of psychological distress. The help that people like Tony offer is a 'talking' therapy aimed at helping the person to sort out their problems. This is a time-consuming option, which is why Tony would have 30 minute appointments rather than the standard eight minutes to see a GP. The benefits for the patients are obvious: a busy GP without the time or the therapeutic training would often have to resort to prescribing a pill to reduce anxiety, which might help in the short term, but does little to cure the cause of the person's problem.

## References

Bower, P. (2002) Primary care mental health workers. Models of working and evidence of effectiveness. *British Journal of General Practice*, **52**, 926–33.

Department of Health (1999) *National Service Framework for Mental Health*. HMSO, London.

George, E., Iveson, C. and Ratner, H. (1999) *Problem to Solution: Brief Therapy with Individuals and Families*, 2nd edn. Brief Therapy Press, London.

Gilbert, P. (2002) *Overcoming Depression: a Self-Help Guide Using Cognitive-Behavioural Techniques*. Robinson, London.

Perris, M. (2003) Psychological therapy in primary care. *Psychoanalytic Psychotherapy*, **17**(1), 18–34.

# CHAPTER 10

# The experience of a practice nurse

*Lindsey Wilkins*

## Editor's introduction

Practices nurses are those people who work in the physical building of a GP practice. Sometimes this is the practice building itself, which may have anything from one to twenty or more GPs, or it may be within a GP-based Health Centre. Unlike District Nurses and Health Visitors, who are employed by the Primary Care Trust/NHS, practice nurses are employed by the GPs, who are themselves independently contracted to the PCT/NHS (there are some exceptions to this, but this is the general structure). This means that practice nurses have a unique employment status compared to the majority of nurses who are employed directly by the NHS. This means that their terms and conditions of employment, annual leave entitlement and study leave support are all subject to the specific contract of employment with individual GP practices. For many practice nurses this is not an issue and most GPs mirror the majority of conditions offered to nurses employed in the NHS. However, some practice nurses do not experience the support that others have come to expect, particularly in terms of annual leave and study leave support. Lindsey's example is of a GP practice that values highly all of its staff – receptionists, practice managers, GPs and practice nurses – and works hard to provide an efficient and first-class service to all of its patients.

The implication of this somewhat unique employment status of the practice nurse is that the roles of different practice nurses can vary enormously, because the individual's role is not dictated by some central PCT line/nurse manager. The role will develop according to the needs of the

GP practice and to some extent the skills of the practice nurse. This will also be influenced to some extent by the size of the GP practice. Thus a practice that has eight or more partners may employ six practices nurses all having a different speciality (e.g. asthma, diabetes, heart failure, smoking cessation, family planning), whilst a practice nurse working in a small one-person practice may well develop generic skills but little in the way of specialist skills or clinics.

Over relatively recent years there has been a developing emphasis on encouraging a larger collection of GPs in one practice with different GPs developing different specialities. These larger practice centres have also fostered the development of different practice nurses, also developing different specialities. This is often driven by the way that government attaches new funding to new services. These moves, together with the changes in legislation that allow experienced nurses with the appropriate qualification to prescribe certain medications, have led to a variety of innovative opportunities for practice nurses.

Like many of the nursing roles in the community the practice nurse works in quite an independent way without the direct support of a team. Many nurses would not feel that they had the experience or competence to undertake this role until they had been qualified for several years. However, as the size of practices increases and they develop into centres of health care, there is far more opportunity to employ 'trainee' practice nurses who are helped to develop the specific skills required to work as a practice nurse. The opportunities for role development have increase greatly in recent years and it is likely that such opportunities will continue as the focus of health care and treatment moves more prominently into the community.

# Practice nurse

## My role

The overall aim of my post is to offer a patient-centred approach to the delivery of nursing care in the general practice setting

Key responsibilities:

- To provide direct access to specialist nursing care
- To undertake health screening, health surveillance and therapeutic interventions within a broad health promotion/public health strategy

■ To support and enable individuals, carers and families to take action to meet their priorities for health

## My typical week

I work at a busy inner city group practice of eight GPs. It is a training practice for student doctors and trainee GPs and serves a practice population of around 10,000 patients. It is situated in an area of socio-economic deprivation. As a training practice, we have GP registrars and medical students, and a variety of nurses and support worker students, all gaining experience in general practice.

Although previously a full-time practice nurse, I now work in practice for two days each week; the other three days a week are spent as Practice Nurse Advisor for Leicester City West Primary Care Trust (PCT). I am fortunate to have a couple of hours on a Monday morning to catch up with paperwork and patients' records. I receive women's cervical smear results from the cytology laboratory and update their computer records, noting the women who need early repeat smears for cervical abnormalities. I refer women who need further investigation to the colposcopy clinic and contact these women to discuss their smear result and reasons for referral. Accurate follow-up for these women is very important, and our team includes administrative support from our chronic disease coordinator, who ensures that women attend for repeat smears on time.

I answer my practice emails and sort out any test results that have come through from the pathology or haematology laboratories. I also check my practice nurse emails – there are often opportunities for study days, meetings or courses that may be of interest. Because our practice is paper-free I will have some practice notes to sort out too. These are electronic messages which are attached to patient records and replace the bits of paper that used to be stuck to hard copies of patient records. The advantage of this is that there is a clear record of actions taken in the patient record. GPs and practice nurses are available for telephone advice requests from patients, and I return these calls before my first patient arrives at the beginning of the morning session. All patient consultations are recorded on the computer. I also need to remember to check the computer telephone advice screen throughout the day to make sure that patients, families or carers do not wait too long for advice.

The practice team meets at coffee time – if we are lucky, there may be a home-made cake to share. I then go back to work, seeing patients of all ages every ten minutes – although I have longer appointment slots for respiratory checks, cervical smears or travel advice. The half hour before lunch is spent making sure that any blood tests, urine tests or cervical smear slides I have taken are ready for collection by the pathology laboratory van, which arrives at about

1:00 p.m. every weekday. This is the time that I can discuss any problems or issues with my GP or practice nurse colleagues. I may need to get in touch with a community nurse, school nurse or health visitor colleague to discuss a patient issue that has arisen during the session. We have a thirty minute lunch break, which we spend together in the staff room. We have regular education meetings for the whole primary health care team, including our District Nurse, Health Visitor and community midwife colleagues when the practice provides lunch and one of the team will give a presentation to the group.

Patients can make appointments to see the practice nurse at any time. The only session we have as a clinic is my chronic obstructive pulmonary disease clinic. This means that the day is full of variety, bearing in mind that patients may make an appointment for one problem but bring other health or social care issues with them that they need to discuss. I will typically see patients for contraceptive advice, blood pressure reviews, asthma checks, cervical smears, weight loss advice, travel immunisations and travel health advice. I have two open appointments every morning and afternoon; this means that I am available for people who need to be seen on that day. These appointments are useful for women who need emergency contraception or who are overdue for their long-acting contraceptive injection.

At the end of the day I make sure I have answered any telephone calls and sorted out any problems that may have come up during the afternoon. I make sure that any specimens are safely packed up and ready for collection the following day and leave the room tidy for a new day tomorrow.

## How I got into this job

I have been a practice nurse since 1989. Before this, I worked as a midwife caring for mothers and babies in a very busy maternity unit. Around this time, GPs were realising that general practice was changing and that if they wanted to deliver high-quality care with an emphasis on health promotion then employing a practice nurse was a priority.

My first job was as a part-time practice nurse in a six-partner practice serving a semi-rural population of 12,000 patients. I was the first practice nurse the practice had employed, so I was lucky enough to be able to develop the role (and myself) to meet the needs of our practice population. In 1990, a new GP contract provided funding for screening clinics to be undertaken by practice nurses. The practice employed another practice nurse who I enjoyed supporting as she developed her practice nurse competencies. By this time I had a special interest in respiratory care and women's health and was able to undertake diploma level courses in these areas. I also attended the first practice nurse course at the then Leicester Polytechnic, which made me realise that there was a lot that I needed and wanted to learn, especially around the politics of health. I undertook a part-time Health Studies degree, which was hard work with two small children but I loved it. At the moment I am busy completing my dissertation for an MA in Applied Health Studies. There is no common entry criterion for practice nursing other than registration with the NMC. GPs are independent contractors and employ their staff, so every practice nurse may have a different job description, different terms and conditions, come from a different nursing background and have a different expectation of the role. However, a considerable amount of funded training and development opportunities is available for practice nurses, and our local university, De Montfort University, offers a practice nurse pathway on a two-year part-time BSc Community Health Nursing degree. As practice nurses we need to recognise the limits of our competence and ask advice or refer the patient to the most appropriate health care professional when we realise that a situation is beyond our skills.

Over the years I combined that first practice nurse post (I stayed there for 12 years) with working in other practices. I was a Nurse Advisor at the Loughborough NHS Walk-In Centre and the Practice Nurse Co-ordinator for the Primary Care Group. I also became a practice nurse clinical supervisor. Nearly five years ago I felt the time was right for a new challenge and started work at my current group practice as a full-time practice nurse. Since becoming the Practice Nurse Advisor I have reduced my time in practice to two days a week. This is ideal for me, because I am not losing touch with the hands-on practice nurse role. Our practice nursing team comprises four practice nurses, a health care assistant and the chronic disease management coordinator. The practice manager and our reception and administrative staff are vital members of the team. We work closely with our Health Visitor, District Nurse and community midwifery colleagues.

## Pleasures, challenges and future directions

I love the variety of my role. Every day in practice is different and brings its own challenges. I see patients of all ages and for lots of different reasons. Practice nursing is about much more than completing a task – a patient may come in to see me to discuss how to lose weight, but the consultation will be about much more than just asking the patient to stand on the scales and recording how many kilograms they weigh. One of the pleasures of this job is that I will be able to see my patients more than once, so I am able to build up relationships with patients, families and carers. The most important quality for a practice nurse to develop is the ability to listen without making judgements about the way people live their lives. Patients believe that nurses have got the time to listen to them and trust us to respond to their health needs – the challenge is being able to do this within the time available to us.

The ongoing changes in primary care present new challenges to how we deliver care in the general practice setting. The new GMS Contract highlighted the importance of skill mix and team working, while the Quality and Outcomes Framework in the contract rewards practices for providing high-quality care. Taking on new roles means that we have to let go of others. We were fortunate to recruit a health care assistant a couple of years ago. This has changed the way that we practise, in that our health care assistant has taken on much of the day-to-day tasks necessary to keep the practice running smoothly, such as ordering supplies, cleaning and decontaminating instruments and organising the collection of specimens. She has undertaken further training at NVQ Level 3 and now runs a smoking cessation clinic in the practice and carries out baseline ECGs for patients newly diagnosed with hypertension. She also runs a daily phlebotomy clinic. We are currently taking on new roles from our District Nurse and Health Visitor colleagues. This means that, together with a practice nurse colleague, I will be carrying out routine childhood immunisation in the future and that our health care assistant will be undertaking an ear care course so that she can gain competencies in ear care.

The changes that reconfiguration of PCTs will mean are yet to become clear, but they are likely to bring new challenges with them. The advent of Practice Based Commissioning will bring individual GP practices into closer working relationships with each other. Practice nurse skills will be in demand as groups of practices work together to meet the needs of their practice populations. It may be that one or two practices have the skills in a specific area, such as sexual health, and could provide this service for a group of practices. I welcome this opportunity for collaborative working, which should lead to more equitable provision of services for patients. The long-term condition agenda is central to practice nursing. Our practice nurse team has skills in the care of patients with diabetes, asthma, coronary heart disease and chronic obstructive pulmonary disease, and is working with patients, carers and families at levels one and two of the long-term conditions triangle. The recent White Paper on community health services underlines the role of primary care and advocates a further shift from the acute to the primary care setting. This will expand the practice nurse role, especially in areas such as first contact care and sexual health. In our practice this is the direction that the practice nurse team has been taking over recent years.

# My typical patient care

## Patient 1

Forty-three-year-old Mr Timmins came to see me recently. He had previously seen the GP about a painful knee and the GP had checked his blood pressure during this consultation. His blood pressure was found to be elevated at 150/92 and the GP had noted that he was overweight, with a BMI of 32. Mr Timmins lives with his partner and they have five young children. He is currently unemployed. I made Mr Timmins welcome and he explained that the GP had asked him to see me to have his blood pressure checked again. We chatted about the changes he had made to his diet. He had cut down on his sugar and fat intake and had increased the amount of fruit and vegetables he was eating. Crisps and chocolate had been banned from the house (his children were now encouraged to have a piece of fruit instead). He had cut his smoking down to five cigarettes a day and aimed to stop. Previously he had tended to drink 30 units of alcohol over Friday and Saturday nights, but had reduced this and aimed to cut down further. He walked the children to school and back every day. He had a family history of heart disease, with his father having developed angina in his fifties and his brother having had a heart attack in his late forties. I took a blood sample to check his lipids, urea and electrolytes and random blood sugar, and arranged for him to bring a urine specimen with him next time for me to test. I checked his blood pressure, which was still raised at 148/98. He was very disappointed that he had actually gained weight despite the changes he had made. After encouraging him to talk me through what he was eating and drinking each day, he told me that he was drinking 1.5 litres of a high-energy glucose drink every day. He had not realised that this drink had a very high sugar content and thought that it was a healthy alternative to the sweet fizzy drinks he had been drinking before. We talked about healthy eating, taking daily exercise, and the importance of smoking cessation, and agreed to meet in another four weeks for a further blood pressure check. He was happy to bring a food diary with him to this appointment. We discussed the possibility of medication to control his blood pressure in the future and arranged an appointment for a baseline ECG prior to his next appointment with me. By taking the time to build up some rapport with Mr Timmins he was relaxed enough to discuss his concerns about his weight and is likely to come back for review.

**Patient 2**

Jenny Davis is a 25-year-old woman who attended for a routine cervical smear. She works as a care assistant in a residential home. After I had greeted her and made her feel welcome she explained that she had never had a smear before and was anxious about the procedure. We talked about the cervical screening programme and she understood why it was important for women to attend for screening. We discussed her menstrual history and the contraception she was currently using. Jenny was taking the contraceptive pill but disclosed that she had a new partner who did not always use condoms. She had noticed some bleeding after sex and some bleeding in between her periods. She had not had any late or missed pills. She had no pain and no vaginal discharge, and did not feel feverish or unwell. Jenny was concerned that she may have been at risk of a sexually transmitted infection (STI). Jenny did not want to go to the Genito-Urinary Medicine (GUM) clinic. We talked about the STIs that we could screen for in the general practice setting and Jenny agreed to have some swabs taken although I advised her that she would need to see her GP about her abnormal bleeding. We discussed possible follow-up if she did have an STI and the need to go to the GUM clinic for further tests and contact tracing. She also understood that I was not screening her for HIV, Hep B or C or syphilis. I explained the procedure and reassured her that she was in control and that we could stop at any time if she became uncomfortable.

I took the smear followed by the swabs; Jenny was surprised that the procedure was much easier than she had thought it would be. I made sure that she understood how she would get the results of her smear and how long it was likely to take. I also made sure we had contact details so that if her swabs showed any infection we could get in touch with her. She was aware that she could ring the practice herself to get the results if she preferred (bearing in mind that we would only contact her if the results showed an infection). We talked about the importance of using condoms, even though she was taking the contraceptive pill and she was happy to take a condom supply with her. I also gave her a GUM clinic card showing their contact details and opening times. She planned to discuss this with her partner and encourage him to visit the clinic for a check-up.

**Patient 3**

Kelly is 11 years old and came with her mother for an asthma check. She lives with her mother and has four younger brothers. Her asthma had been more of a problem recently, despite taking her preventer inhaler twice a day. The main trigger appeared to be exercise. Her mother could hear her coughing several nights a week. Her mother also said her breathing was very noisy at night and that she sounded as though she was snoring. I chatted to Kelly about how much she had grown in the last year while measuring her height and checking her peak expiratory flow rate. I had noticed that Kelly looked tired and was mouth breathing and sniffing throughout the consultation. Kelly told me that she was unhappy at school, other children were teasing her about her constant sniffing and blocked up nose. She couldn't take a very active part in PE and games sessions because exercise made her cough and wheeze. She felt tired during the day. Together, Kelly and I went through how she was using her preventer and reliever inhalers. Her inhaler technique was poor, as she was finding the metered dose inhaler difficult to use effectively. We changed these to a breath-actuated device which she thought she would be happy to use after I demonstrated the correct technique. I also got the doctor to prescribe a once-daily nasal spray and showed Kelly how to use it. She agreed to continue to use her preventer twice a day and to use the reliever when necessary and before exercise. I reassured Kelly and her mother that I would speak to the school nurse about the difficulties at school and encouraged Kelly's mother to discuss the issue with Kelly's teacher. When I saw Kelly again four weeks later, she looked much better. Her nasal symptoms had cleared up, she was no longer mouth breathing and she could sleep through the night. Kelly said that life at school was much easier – the nasal spray and regular use of the preventer inhaler had transformed her into a girl who could breathe comfortably through her nose, enjoy her food, sleep through the night and enjoy PE and games lessons. The problems at school had been tackled with the support of the school nurse and teachers and Kelly was much more confident and happy at school.

## Student nurses on placement

Learning aim:

- To understand the contribution that practice nursing makes to the delivery of high-quality patient care in a general practice setting

Learning objectives:

- to become familiar with the practice profile for Group Practice
- to gain insight into the day-to-day running of a general practice by spending time with a receptionist, the chronic disease management coordinator, the health care assistant and at least one GP
- to spend time with each of the practice nurses at the practice in order to gain insight into the breadth and depth of the practice nursing role
  I would expect a student nurse on placement with us to:
- be neat and tidy in appearance (not necessary to wear a uniform unless they prefer to)
- arrive at the practice on time
- have made him/herself familiar with the practice area so that they have some idea of the needs of our practice population
- be friendly and polite to our patients
- have plenty of questions to ask team members

Student nurses on placement at our practice should bring a packed lunch with them (although there are shops close by if they forget!). Coffee and tea are provided. It would be a good idea for them to spend their lunch breaks at the practice so that they get to know the whole team. They will be made very welcome. Buses leave the city centre regularly and stop very near to the practice. There is on-street car parking available.

## Editor's comments

If you have already been on your community placement and managed to work with a practice nurse, how did it compare with Lindsey's description? Is this a role that you can see yourself doing in a few years' time, or would you miss the 'hustle and bustle' of ward work? From the perspective of the patient, the practice nurse has the potential to become a key figure in the coordination and maintenance of care continuity particularly for patients with chronic conditions. It is a very rewarding part of nursing to be able to follow the same patient through their care and treatment, often spanning a number of years: and for the patient it is very reassuring to see the same face on different visits.

## References

Crisp, N. (2005) *Commissioning a Patient Led NHS*. Department of Health, London.

Department of Health (2002) *Liberating the Talents: Helping Primary Care Trusts to deliver the NHS Plan*. Department of Health, London.

Department of Health (2004a) *The NHS Improvement Plan: Putting People at the Heart of Public Services*. Department of Health, London.

Department of Health (2004b) *Choosing Health – Making Healthy Choices Easier*. Department of Health, London.

Department of Health (2004c) *The National Health Service (General Medical Services Contracts) Regulations*. HMSO, London.

Department of Health (2004d) *Practice Based Commissioning: Promoting Clinical Engagement*. Department of Health, London.

Department of Health (2005a) *Supporting People with Long Term Conditions: An NHS and Social Care Model to Support Local Innovation and Integration*. Department of Health, London.

Department of Health (2005b) *Supporting People with Long Term Conditions: Liberating the Talents of Nurses Who Care for People with Long Term Conditions*. Department of Health, London.

Department of Health (2006) *Our Health, Our Care, Our Say: a New Direction in Community Services*. Department of Health, London.

# CHAPTER 11

# The experience of practice management

*Pat Brookhouse*

## Editor's introduction

This chapter contains an account by Pat Brookhouse, who is the only contributor to this book (apart from Nancy, in Chapter 1), who is not a clinician. You are unlikely to have a placement with the practice manager. You may spend an hour or so with some of the administrative staff, but it is quite difficult to fully appreciate the impact that such roles have upon direct patient care. As you read Pat's account, make sure you translate her actions into the effects that they have on patient care. Often as clinical practitioners we evaluate the quality of the patient's experience as a function of the care that we directly give. However, this is a very superficial perspective. If you talk to any patient, or you have the experience of being a patient, then you will realise that there is a lot more affecting the quality of care than what happens inside the consulting room.

The variety of health care that currently occurs in general practices has increased over the years, and some of the larger surgeries resemble small hospitals in the specialities and resources that they offer. This variety is likely to continue to increase, as government initiatives seem to be encouraging primary care to take a far more interventionist approach to treatment than currently occurs. These developments obviously need the involvement of the clinician to deliver the services, but equally importantly they need the management skills of people like Pat to coordinate all the services that are so vital to the delivery of primary care services.

# Practice management

## Introduction

Overall aims of the post:

- To lead the strategic and operational management of the practice in the delivery of primary care services to the practice population
- To work, in conjunction with the partners, to ensure the viability of the practice as a business
- As a GP Trainer (non-clinical), to participate in the Leicester Deanery Vocational Training Scheme for GP Registrars
- To establish develop and maintain effective working relationships with Leicester City West Primary Care Trust, voluntary agencies and other service providers
  Key responsibilities:
- Strategic planning
- Recruitment and management of all practice staff: reception, administrative and nursing
- Stability of partnership: recruitment of partners and GPs
- Practice finance: management of accounts, payroll, superannuation, PMS contract, enhanced services and Quality and Outcomes Framework
- Practice-based commissioning
- Operational management
- Service provision
- Complaints, significant events, critical incidents
- Premises: cleaning, maintenance and repairs
- Information technology
- Health and safety
- Clinical governance
- Community staff: District Nurses, Health Visitors, midwives, practice therapists
- Communication
- Liaison with LCW PCT, voluntary agencies and local groups
- GP trainer/education

## How I got into this job

Prior to joining the practice I worked in the pharmacy department at the local hospital, initially as an invoice clerk on a six-week rolling contract. Eight years later, given the opportunity, support and encouragement of the Pharmacy Manager, I completed my Postgraduate Certificate and Diploma in Health Services Management and attained the dizzy heights of Administrative Services Manager, responsible for the purchase (expenditure of £2.5 million), receipt and delivery of drugs to other hospitals bought on behalf of the South Trent Consortium. I had, realistically, progressed as far as I could within pharmacy, and having achieved my postgraduate qualification was eager to progress.

I spotted an advert in the local paper for a practice manager at a local GP's Group Practice. At the time no particular qualifications were asked for, but today most new recruits to the profession have a either a postgraduate qualification or a recognised qualification such as the Diploma in Primary Care Management awarded by the Association of Medical Secretaries, Practice Managers Administrators and Receptionists (AMSPAR), along with proven experience of motivating people and managing change.

Practice management today is recognised as a profession, and the Institute of Healthcare Management is piloting a one-year Vocational Training Scheme for newly appointed practice managers or anyone seeking to move into a managerial position from an administrative post by working their way through a series of competencies based on the NHS Skills and Knowledge Framework to achieve an agreed standard.

I applied for the job, and was asked to attend for interview and to prepare a presentation on 'Staff Performance'. The title should have told me something about the difficulties in the practice at that time, but undaunted I delivered it to an interview panel of seven partners, one practice nurse, one (hostile) reception manager and a representative from the then Health Authority. It must have gone well, as I was offered the job. I have to say that I knew next to nothing about primary care or general practice in particular when I started, but again was lucky enough to have an extremely supportive and go-ahead bunch of young GPs keen (although this enthusiasm was not shared by some of the other staff) to develop and change the way in which services were delivered and to tackle the staff issues, some of which were related to the organisation and structure of the practice.

## What does the role entail?

Being a practice manager in a seven-partner teaching and training practice serving 10,000 patients is a bit like looking after a large diverse family all living under the same roof, with much the same needs, wants and expectations. It is the manager who provides the leadership required to make any team a cohesive unit by bringing vision, objectivity and fairness to the management of different disciplines. The practice is a democracy in which all levels of staff are represented on working parties and whose opinions and ideas are listened to, considered and implemented. The practice is committed to promoting and maintaining a practice culture where staff are encouraged to continually develop new skills, respond to the changing environment and be a valued member of the team. There is an opportunity to develop skills and undertake further training to NVQ or postgraduate qualification level for administrators, receptionists and health care assistants, whilst practice nurses are encouraged to enhance their skills in specialist roles or consider degree- or masters-level qualifications.

We are a teaching practice for fourth-year medical undergraduates, who are with us for an eight-week placements. They sit in with the doctors and begin to consult with patients, taking histories and starting to think about the structure of the consultation, diagnoses, management plans and the role of the patient in the consultation by asking for and considering their ideas, concerns and expectations. They have two assessments during this time, the second being a final assessment which, if successful, will see them on to the next stage of their training. Our practice has three GP trainers. Doctors who decide to become GPs have to undertake a further year's training in General Practice and be signed off by their trainer against a set of national criteria. We can have up to four Registrars at any one time and I act as their educational supervisor. I organise and give tutorials in practice management: finance, practice accounts, employment law, complaints, practice-based commissioning and other non-clinical training needs identified in their personal development plans.

I have full responsibility for the management of the organisation. I can make a range of decisions without reference to the partners. These include, within previously agreed budgets:

- Recruitment of all staff
- Replacement of staff
- Changes to the organisational structure
- Training and development of staff
- Pay awards
- Recommendations on policy and procedures
- Authorisation of expenditure on furniture and equipment
- Premises repairs and maintenance

I organise my own time. I can mix and match my time in the practice and the work I need to complete to suit, but generally my week begins at 8:00 a.m. each Monday morning with a 'start the week meeting', with all doctors, GP Registrars and my reception manager meeting over coffee to consider the week ahead and the monthly doctor rota. The reception manager advises on who is in or on annual leave and on appointment availability for the week ahead, and we adjust the number of available routine appointments if we are unable to meet the 48/24 hour access requirements. This is an opportunity to look at any gaps or shortfalls in the rota for the coming month and to juggle who's in and out, swap sessions and on-calls etc., or agree if we need locums. If there is any time left, anyone can raise an issue that needs a quick decision or a problem that can be easily resolved. Half an hour later we all disperse to our desks, to meet later over coffee or lunch.

No two days or weeks are the same, but I try to divide my day into two halves. In the mornings I start by opening post, checking emails, emptying my pigeon hole and dealing with any queries from staff, PCT, suppliers or general enquiries. Although I do not spend any regular time in reception, there are occasions when it is particularly busy, so I cover coffee breaks or staff sickness. When I man the phones or deal with patients at reception I remind myself what a difficult job the receptionists have, dealing with the requirements and expectations of patients and doctors, and how well they do it.

Coffee time for the GPs is 10:45 a.m. and usually they will all manage to get together. This is a time for bringing up any clinical questions that have arisen from morning surgery or any operational problems that have arisen. I try to join them at this time. Late morning each day brings a variety of work, such as sorting invoices, replying to correspondence, preparing wages, writing cheques, ordering supplies, and preparing agendas for and minutes of meetings. Over the past year we have had a four-roomed extension added to the existing building. This consisted of three consulting rooms and a preparation room added as an annex to the treatment room. Most mornings have seen me liaising with the builders, organising out-of-bounds areas within the practice and shuffling clinics. Minor surgery sessions had to be cancelled whilst the builders knocked through into the treatment room, creating lots of dust and dirt.

Most lunchtimes are taken up with meetings of one sort or another. As practice manager I attend the majority of them. This is the core part of the role: providing leadership and direction to all. Good communication and information ensure that staff and patients know what is happening in the practice. Awaydays and partnership meetings deal with the long-term planning and strategy for the practice in terms of staff, finance, workload, and implementation of Government policies working with the Primary Care Trust. A team meeting allows all staff to come together over lunch, which the practice provides. An early morning trip to Marks & Spencer for a selection of goodies for lunch is a great way of ensuring a good turnout. These meetings include a mixture of educational updates, results of audits, new guidelines, or a general 'what's happening' in the practice at the moment briefing. They meetings give staff the opportunity to catch up with each other on a social level too. Clinical governance agendas included complaint monitoring and any significant events or critical incidents. Other meetings, such as health and safety, IT, training, and research and development, take place quarterly.

Practice staff get together monthly to discuss any issues relevant to their working group. I see the reception manager and the lead practice nurse weekly over a working lunch.

All of our community staff, including District Nurses, Health Visitors, midwives and practice therapist, have on-site office accommodation and I try to catch up with them on a weekly basis as well as meeting with them more formally.

The afternoon is a time when I can close the door and consider the strategic direction of the practice, work on projects, new developments and appraisals, talk to individual GPs, and build and improve relationships with our PMS contract and Quality and Outcome Framework (QOF). Some of the most recent projects have included:

- Agenda for change: revisiting job descriptions and pay policy
- Review of GP Registrars' working schedules within the practice in the light of new guidance
- Review of policy and procedures in preparation for the quality review undertaken by the PCT
- Practice-based commissioning: completion of local delivery plans
- Enhanced services: service specification and budget setting
- Preparation for new intake of GP Registrars
- Protected time to talk to staff
- Appraisals

I meet a variety of people over the course of the week outside of practice staff. A typical week sees me meeting with the newly appointed Community Matrons to give them an overview of life in practice, to understand their role and to explore how we can work together to benefit patients and save time and money. I meet with the Director of Primary Care at the PCT to discuss our annual budget and payments for enhanced services and the flu campaign. I have visits from people running local self-help groups or voluntary agencies wanting me to advise on the latest project or eager to advise us of new groups that have been formed.

## Our extended family

And then there are the patients: 10,000 of them – our extended family! We work in the inner city providing services to a deprived population. We get to know them well as individuals and family units. We come to understand their history and the complicated lives that some of them lead. There are higher than average incidences of diabetes, hypertension, smoking and asthma. The numbers of single and teenage mothers continue to rise, bringing the associated problems of depression, mental health and sexually transmitted diseases, along with child and adolescent behavioural problems. Our patients do appreciate the time and effort that the team put in to providing the level of service that we, as patients, would want from our own practices, by dealing with patients in a courteous, friendly and efficient manner. Our patient satisfaction surveys reflect the regard in which the patients hold the practice. Nevertheless, things do go wrong from time to time and I deal with and respond to complaints from patients, learn from the issues and continually review what we do to ensure that systems run smoothly. On occasion, if there is a complaint of a clinical nature that cannot be resolved by a letter, both the doctor and I will meet the patient to discuss the issues in order to resolve them as quickly and amicably as possible.

## The way forward

This year I have undertaken the Postgraduate Certificate in Medical Education, which will allow me to be a GP trainer in the practice. This will mean a complete overhaul of my working week once I have passed. I will be assigned my own GP Registrar and will work with them to formulate a personal development and learning plan and improve their consulting skills. I will be involved in debriefing GP Registrars at the end of morning surgeries and participating in the provision of tutorials to GP Registrars in the non-clinical aspects of practice management and life.

I undertake some work with the Leicester Deanery in the revalidation of training practices. Some weeks will find me visiting training practices with established GP trainers. I review the individual practice arrangements for training registrars, whilst the GP will look at the teaching logs and videos of the GP trainers. Most practices pass with flying colours and it is good to spend a morning with other practice managers and come away with lots of new ideas for your own practice.

I have been fortunate enough to have been asked to work with several practices and PCTs on a consultancy basis, and for the past three years I have been working with another city PCT for two days a week looking after three directly managed practices, acting as a mentor to the practice managers, and offering expertise and advice as required.

Variety is the spice of life, and this job certainly affords it. As well as leading a successful, innovative, forward-thinking practice, most of my job satisfaction comes from giving staff the opportunity to develop their skills. We take a number of reception and administrative staff from the area we serve. Their educational achievement in school has in some cases been low, but given the challenge of employment and time at college to enable them to gain a qualification that may lead to a better job and a good salary, all of them find success – sometimes for the first time in their life. This does wonders for their self-esteem, self-worth and self-confidence. It is rewarding to see newly qualified doctors, who have spent a lot of time in hospital, getting to grips with some of our more challenging patients on their own turf and beginning to see the social and economic dilemmas that our patients have to deal with.

Managing change is what practice managers do best. Fundholding, new GMS/PMS contracts, changes to out-of-hours services, computerisation, Health Authorities, and the evolution of Strategic Health Authorities and Primary Care Trusts are all examples of the numerous changes that taken place over the past ten years.

The challenges for the future are likely to be:

- Wider patient choice
- Implementation of advanced IT systems, e.g. choosing and booking electronic referrals
- Increased number of private providers of service and the implications for primary care
- Improved access to GPs and health professionals
- Practice-based commissioning
- Expansion of the Quality and Outcome Framework
- Ensuring that practices have the skills and competencies to deliver what is needed
- Collaborative working with other practices
- Changes to patient registration and practice areas

General practice will continue to offer patients what they want and value. Nine out of ten people in a recent survey of 10,000 people thought that it was important to be treated by a doctor who knows them and their family, who listens, and who explains treatments in a way that they can understand.

Whatever the challenges, practice managers will continue to do what they do best: implement change, continue to be proactive, face up to the responsibilities of the job and deliver whatever is asked of them.

## Editor's comments

I think you will have been surprised at the amount of work and the responsibility that is involved in Pat's role. Whilst she does not have direct clinical contact, her work does have a very real impact on the care that patients receive. First impressions are very important for most of us when visiting the GP. The way in which the receptionist greets us, the type of chairs we sit on, the furnishing, the appointment system etc. all affect the way we feel before we get in to see the doctor. It is the practice manager who leads this team and sets the standard for the practice. Doctors and nurses are clinicians, and hopefully skilled and expert in their speciality, but they are not normally good managers and administrators: this is the expertise of the practice manager. Health care does not just happen – it needs to be managed and planned. Teamwork is more than a collection of clinicians. Pat is fortunate to be working in a practice in which the partners (GPs) have respect for all the other staff that work in their practice. This atmosphere of respect is then communicated to all the patients that visit the surgery. This is an extremely important point for all clinicians to learn: health care works as a team, and how we get treated is usually reflected in the way we treat others.

# CHAPTER 12

# A student's experience

*Sarah Hudson*

## Editor's introduction

You will see as you read Sarah's account that she takes a very mature approach to her learning. She puts herself firmly in charge of her learning and actively gets involved with the team, her patients and the community experience in general. This is a perfect example of how to get the most out of any of your placements, but particularly the community placement. In your ward placements you can learn a lot by simply standing, watching and helping out. In the community it is a little different: if you stand back and don't show interest and enthusiasm, then you will find yourself becoming easily bored. Sarah's community experience was in her third year. She had an orientation placement earlier in her training, but this was her main community experience. Her mentors and the university would expect a student at this stage of training to be capable of undertaking a degree of supervised yet independent responsibility for patient care, and Sarah's account demonstrates this well.

## Student's progress

I was asked to write this chapter mid-way through my third year as a student nurse at De Montfort University, Leicester. I began my training at the age of 35, prior to which I had been employed as a dental nurse and latterly as a team leader and venepuncturist for the National Blood Service. I feel that there have been many advantages to beginning nursing later in life, and believe that life experience and the confidence brought about by surviving life's challenges are the most valuable things that anyone can take forward into practice.

## My placement

My community experience was the first placement of my third year of training. When I received notification of my upcoming placement I was very pleased, as it was the health centre I had requested, close to my home address, in an area I knew well. The district nursing team based there covered three medical practices within the county of Leicestershire. The placement, which was only two two months ago as I write this account, seems like a distant memory, probably because it was so different and I am now back on familiar territory in the hospital environment.

I tried to approach the placement with an open mind, but if I'm honest I expected it to be very 'slow', particularly after my previous placement, which was in a cardiac intensive care unit. I was looking forward to the regular hours of 8:30 a.m.–5:00 p.m. and having a regular shift pattern, and as the health centre was close to home the opportunity to be able to go home for lunch seemed attractive. I felt all the usual feelings of apprehension when starting a new placement. Would I fit in? Would my allocated mentor be supportive? What would the patients be like? I was also aware that for the last three weeks of the placement I would be expected to go out in the community, visit patients on my own and manage my own caseload of patients, without the familiar consolation that there was a qualified nurse just behind me, or at least somewhere outside the curtains! I was concerned that I didn't have much experience of doing dressings and had a real fear of getting lost and arriving late at patients' homes, despite being quite close to home!

I contacted my allocated mentor approximately two weeks before the date I was due to start my placement in order to introduce myself, confirm that they had received notification from the university and obtain my hours of work. On my first day I arrived in uniform at 8:30 a.m. I was introduced to everyone and shown around the health centre. I was immediately made to feel very welcome. My personalised student planner was already on the noticeboard and my first week had been planned.

The district nursing team met each morning at 8:30 a.m., before going out on visits, to plan their day's work, collect supplies, discuss any concerns relating to patient care, and have a nice cup of coffee and a quick chat! The community nurses and auxiliaries had their own lists of patients and were responsible for their own planners. Patients were allocated to their named nurse by the charge nurse based on the patient's initial assessment; this allocation depended on the health centre at which the patient was registered and the reason for referral. This informal 'handover' took place again after lunch at 2:00 p.m., when outstanding paperwork and any telephone referrals could be done. These meetings certainly promoted effective team working and required the nurses to utilise their communication skills.

The first few weeks of my placement were spent primarily as an observer, going out with various community nurses and getting to know them, their varying roles and their patients, while familiarising myself with the community routines and various tasks that were carried out. As time progressed I was soon able to complete some of the work and relevant documentation myself while being guided and observed. This gradually built up until I was ready to competently and confidently take on my own small caseload of approximately 15 patients during my 'delegated care' period .

## Nursing in the community

Nursing in the community is different from nursing in the hospital setting in many ways, but the main difference is obviously that you are going into a patient's home environment to deliver care, instead of them coming into 'your' (hospital) environment; you are a guest and the onus of control is with the patient. You must ask permission to sit down, to go and wash your hands in their kitchen or bathroom, or to put your supplies on their table or chair. This is especially true until a relationship and mutual trust have been established.

When the patient is assessed in their own home, it is easier to see the full picture of their life/lifestyle and therefore plan truly individualised care based on a full holistic assessment of their needs. The team I worked with did not use the core, pre-printed care plans seen on the hospital wards. You actually had to write them yourself, which made the care far more patient-centred and provided valuable experience.

The assignment set for the community module partly involved collecting demographic and epidemiological data relating to the area in which I was placed. This enabled factors such as housing, age, ethnicity, social deprivation and employment to be seen in relation to patients' health. Health and social problems affecting the local community and the initiatives aimed at tackling these problems were also identified. This knowledge of available services could then be communicated to patients and their families, thus promoting health. Government legislation, although very complex, was also studied for my assignment, and this allowed me to see how it impacts on the health of individuals within the community.

Working within the community team enabled me to learn many new skills and helped consolidate the skills I had already acquired. The cases in which I was involved included wound care, particularly leg ulcers, and some diabetic patients who had tissue viability problems; I found the myriad of different dressings that were available amazing. Then there was post-operative care: patients discharged from hospital were often referred to have sutures or clips removed, and it was interesting to see the other side of filling in discharge letters while working on the wards. Homebound patients with various conditions required blood samples to be taken, and others needing prompting to take their medication or help with administering medications such as eye drops or insulin. Flu and pneumonia vaccinations in the winter months play a big part in the community nurse's day. The majority of the District Nurse's workload is taken up with older people who require these vaccinations, so there is plenty of opportunity to brush up on your injection technique. Catheter care and continence assessments were also commonplace, as well as palliative care for the terminally ill. The community nurses also ran clinics once a week for those who were able to come in for their treatment, and I was able to assist during these clinics. They included ear syringing, leg ulcer and general wound care clinics.

Home to some patients is a residential home, and the district nursing team also provided care in this environment. As part of my delegated care I had some patients to visit in residential care; indeed, the patient I chose for my assignment case study was one of them. Good communication, both verbal and written, is required to provide care staff and other health professionals with the information they need to ensure continuity of appropriate care, even when the nurse is not there.

The team was involved in making referrals to other health care professionals, such as social workers. Many patients required equipment or modifications to their homes to allow them to carry out their activities of living safely, while others benefited from a package of care to allow them to remain in their own homes. My placement enabled me to see various options available and to be involved in the referral process, as well as showing me the importance of collaborative care.

The Primary Care Team was involved not only with their patients but also with the family and friends of these patients; the provision of education and support enabled them to continue contributing quality care to the patients in their own homes, preventing potential hospital admissions. I found that when visiting patients and chatting to them and their families there were many education opportunities to seize upon, and much information can be gathered from 'informal' conversation.

The delegated care period during the last three weeks of my placement enabled me to develop my time management skills and helped me learn to prioritise my care; I had a list of patients to visit during the day and had to decide who to see first, and I also had to ensure that I had the correct supplies with me to enable the task to be carried out properly. It was wonderful, even though it was initially a little daunting, to be able to go out and make my own decisions about patient care. Obviously, care plans were in place to guide me, but I was able to evaluate these and change them if I thought it necessary. It certainly helped build my confidence when I fed back my decisions to the team later in the day and they agreed with my actions!

When nursing in the community, regular visits to the same patient (sometimes as often as daily) can seem repetitive, especially when, as a student, you are not there to see the beginning and the end of their treatment. However, I can see that it must be very rewarding to see your patient discharged from care and fully healed after suffering from long-term conditions such as leg ulcers. It was interesting to see photographs of leg ulcers before and after District Nurse interventions, often showing remarkable improvements. Due to the often long-term nature of the patients' needs it is possible to build up close, trusting relationships with patients, and they may come to see you as their friend, not just their nurse.

## Tips for student nurses on community placement

- Contact your placement a couple of weeks before your start date to make sure they are expecting you and to obtain your off-duty and uniform requirements. It may be necessary to inform them if you do not have your own transport.
- If you do have access to your own transport, check with your insurance company whether or not you are covered for business use; some policies automatically cover you and some don't.
- Start your assignment early and ensure that your mentor is aware of the assessment requirements so that appropriate support may be given.
- Don't just watch when out on visits: ask questions and get involved in the patient's care as much as possible. Be assertive and say what you want to achieve – I found that I learned more by doing than by watching!
- Work the full variety of shifts, including weekends and nights, as often a wider area of the region is covered and you will see different cases out of your usual area.
- Remember to maintain patient confidentiality, as sometimes you will be treating people who live in the same street and questions are often asked by neighbours! Also take care when carrying confidential information around in your car.
- Be proactive and responsible for your own learning. Arrange to spend time in as many different areas as possible. I arranged time with the practice nurse, a funeral director, a community occupational therapist and a community psychiatric nurse, and spent time at the local hospice and with the intermediate care team.
- Work with as many different staff members as possible, from the auxiliaries to the sister; you will see role variations, thus maximising your experience.

- Answer the telephone while in the office to gain experience liaising with the MDT and with patients and their families.
- Regularly discuss your progress. This helps build confidence if all is going well, but also enables any problems that should arise to be addressed early enough for them to be resolved easily.
- Get to know the area and find out what services the local community has to offer your patients and their families.
- Be organised when you visit patients; write your itinerary in a diary and plan your route in advance; take an A–Z street map and ensure that you have everything with you that you will need. Remember that there is no treatment room to go to if you forget something.
- Keep a note of your mileage – you may be able to claim your fuel expenses back; depending on where you are placed mileage could be quite high during your delegated care period.
- Try to find out as much as you can about your patient and their condition before you arrive.
- Make sure you have the telephone number of your mentor programmed into your mobile phone just in case you need advice while with a patient. Make sure your mobile is fully charged so that you can be contacted if necessary.
- Be aware that not all patients live in the same conditions that you do! Carrying out an aseptic technique is not as easy as it is in a hospital, especially when the patient insists on having the dog in the room!
- Make sure your supplies include a tube of alcohol gel for your hands!

As I reflect on my community experience I feel that the skills that I have acquired will be invaluable as I continue down the pathway towards my qualification and on into my nursing career; certainly on my current medical placement, I have felt far more confident when faced with wound dressings and it is nice to know what is out there for patients when they are discharged from hospital. Due to the close working relationships of the community team I have made some good friends who I see socially on a regular basis, and although I may not consider community nursing as my first position on qualifying, I may consider it later on in my career. I enjoyed the experience far more than I expected to, and since I have left I have missed not only the staff but the patients too; some of them have left lasting impressions on me that I shall never forget.

## Editor's comments

You will see from Sarah's account that her community experience was far more than just finding out what the District Nurse did. She learned valuable nursing skills concerned with wound care, communication, patient education, giving injections and taking blood pressure, and many more of the 'softer' skills. In addition to that, she learned to take responsibility for patient care and she learned some of the skills of managing care and decision making without the reassurance of a qualified nurse at the end of the ward. These are tremendous confidence-building activities that are an essential quality of the qualified nurse. At the same time, she gained a real empathy for patients' holistic needs and circumstances, integrating concepts such as social class, government policy, and needs analysis into the realities of nursing practice.

# Index

active learning 19
advice for students 14–16
assessment of patients 23–4, 45
   palliative care 58
   student nurse's view 117
asthma 102–3
asylum seekers 64–71
   illnesses 68–9
   patient care 68–9

blood pressure 100–1
Brookhouse, Pat 106–14
   background 107–8

career structure 67
care plan 36
case histories
   Lilly 59–60
   Marie 69
   Peter 26–8
cervical screening 101–2
children
   child protection 77–8
   Health Visitor 72–82
   palliative care 53–63
children's community nurse specialist 52–63
   research project 54
   responsibilities 53
   working week 54–5
Clements, Ann 33–40
   background 34
clinic 10
communication
   non-verbal 2
   Parkinson's disease 1
communication skills
   community health care assistant 35

   District Nurse 24
community care 5–6
community health care assistant 33–40
   change in role 39–40
   job satisfaction 39–40
   journey planning 36
   in patient's home 36–7
   role 35–6
   sense of humour 37
   skills 35
   training 38
   travel 37
   working week 35–6
community nursing
   apprehensions 10
   career choice 9
   compared with hospital 117–19
   comparison with family life 42
   de-skilling myth 14–15
   expectations 8–10
   perceptions of 9
community practice teacher *see* District
   Nurse

death, support during 27–8
depression 83, 90–1
de-skilling myth 14
diabetic patients 10
discharge, planning 26
District Nurse 18–31, 41–50
   assessment of patients 23–4
   caseload 24–8, 45
   challenges 47–8
   developments in role of 29–30
   job requirements 46
   job satisfaction 18, 47
   leader 19